THE SOUND OF HOPE

THE SOUND OF
HOPE

Recognizing, Coping with, and Treating Your Child's
AUDITORY PROCESSING DISORDER

Lois Kam Heymann, MA, CCC-SLP

WITH A FOREWORD BY
Rosie O'Donnell

BALLANTINE BOOKS / NEW YORK

The Sound of Hope is a work of nonfiction, but with the exception of
Rosie O'Donnell's family, the individual children and families described are
composite portraits, and all names have been changed.

As of press time, the URLs displayed in this book link or refer to existing
websites on the Internet. Random House, Inc., is not responsible for, and
should not be deemed to endorse or recommend, any website other than
its own or any content available on the Internet (including without limitation
at any website, blog page, information page) that is not created by Random House.
The author, similarly, cannot be responsible for third-party material.

Published in the United States by Ballantine Books, an imprint of
The Random House Publishing Group, a division of Random House, Inc., New York.

BALLANTINE and colophon are registered trademarks of Random House, Inc.

LIBRARY OF CONGRESS CATALOGING-IN-PUBLICATION DATA
Heymann, Lois Kam.
The sound of hope : recognizing, coping with, and treating your child's auditory
processing disorder / Lois Kam Heymann ; with a foreword by Rosie O'Donnell.
p. cm.
Includes bibliographical references and index.
ISBN 978–0-345–51218–5 (hardcover : alk. paper)
eBook ISBN 978-0-345-51218-5
1. Word deafness in children—Popular works.   I. O'Donnell, Rosie.   II. Title.
RF291.5.C45H49 2010
618.920978—dc22   2010002090

PRINTED IN THE UNITED STATES OF AMERICA

www.ballantinebooks.com

2 4 6 8 9 7 5 3 1

FIRST EDITION

Book design by Casey Hampton

There are two lasting bequests we can hope to give our children.
One of these is roots, the other, wings.
—Hodding Carter II

This book is dedicated to the many wonderful parents and
children I have worked with over the years and
who have taught me so much.

CONTENTS

PART 3: TREATING APD THROUGH SKILL BUILDING

FOREWORD

My two boys, Blake and Parker, have been getting their hair cut at the same barbershop and by the same barber, Nick, for almost their whole lives. For years now they've each sat down in the chair and smiled up at Nick as he snaps a crisp white sheet in the air and settles it around their shoulders. Familiar sounds fill the place: customers and barbers talking and walking around, piped-in music from the mall outside, snipping scissors, and humming electric razors. A lunch of chili cheese fries at Johnny Rockets after the haircut has always made the day special.

When Blake was about to enter the first grade, he and I went off to find Nick. Blake's hair had grown quite long over the summer, and I was a little worried about how he'd handle the change back to short hair. Compared with Parker, Chelsea, and our youngest, Vivienne, Blakey doesn't really do change so well.

"How do you want it, honey?" I asked. "A crew cut like Parker? Just a trim? What?"

No matter how I phrased it, Blake gave me the same sort of

answer: "A little haircut." I knew from recent experience that if I
pressed him for detail, I could count on what had become his ul-
timate answer to just about every question: "I dunno."

"How do you want it, Blakey?"

"A haircut."

"Yeah, but what kind of haircut?"

"I dunno."

"You want to leave it long? A trim?"

"No, like a little haircut."

"Okay, but how short?"

"I dunno. A little haircut."

At first, I chalked his vagueness up to distraction or simply not
caring all that much. But then Blake seemed frustrated that he
was not able to be clear with me or with Nick about what exactly
he wanted. We didn't have all day, so Nick patted Blake's head,
went to work, and gave Blake a crew cut like the one he'd been
giving Parker for years. I thought it was cute; my partner, Kelli,
thought it was cute; Nick thought it was cute. Blake didn't have
much to say about it right there in the barber chair. He seemed
fine with it. Case closed. Off to Johnny Rockets.

But the next day, we were driving home from school and
Blake was belted into the seat behind me. I asked him if anyone
at school had mentioned his new haircut. He *exploded*! My
adorable son, a kid of so few words but such deep feelings, started
screaming. "I told you not a haircut, and you did me a haircut, not
a trim!" He was beside himself—absolutely melting down. I
couldn't follow what he was saying exactly in words, but the emotions were raw and real and just broke my heart.

I pulled over, got out of the car, opened his door, and took him
in my arms. "Honey, I'm sorry," I said. "I am so sorry. I did not
understand what you wanted, Blakey. I'm very sorry."

"I want my long hair," he said, tears streaming down his face.

"You will never have to get a short haircut ever again," I told him. "I promise you." It took him ten minutes to calm down.

When Blake first came into our lives he was the happiest baby I'd ever seen. I know every mother says that, but he was just beautiful and everybody said so. As an infant, he cooed and smiled and his clothes were always wet with drool. Adorable. As a toddler, he continued to coo—he didn't make sounds that seemed like words. I look back now at the videos we shot during vacations and birthdays when Blake was nearing age three and wonder how we made any sense of what little he did say.

When Blake was three and a half, a friend of ours suggested we get him evaluated by a speech pathologist. The tests said he was perfectly intelligent but was having trouble making and saying words clearly compared with other kids his age. At the speech pathologist's suggestion, Blake had regular speech therapy for the next year. The sessions helped him shape his mouth to make certain sounds that had eluded him, but finding the words in the first place was still difficult for him. As he grew in intelligence and the world around him grew more complicated, Blake was increasingly less happy, more frustrated, and angrier than Kelli and I ever would have believed that sweetly smiling baby could become. When life threw him a curve, as it does for kids at any age, Blake simply didn't have the vocabulary available to express what was wrong, how he felt, or what he needed. "Where's my happy Blakey?" I'd ask him after the umpteenth misunderstanding climaxed in yelling and tears.

Your family's routine sometimes can make it difficult to spot problems with your kids as they grow. But Blake's haircut meltdown was just the latest in a series of misunderstandings, mixed messages, and miscommunications that were increasingly making him angry. These incidents were upsetting for us and just heartbreaking for Blake. He had so many things to share but no

way to share them. It was like the words were stuck inside him—
he couldn't find the way to get them out.

The challenge of using words—understanding them and ar-
ticulating them—just seemed insurmountable to him. Once, for
instance, Blake and Vivienne raced back to our house to tell us
about a family of ducks they had seen swimming nearby. Older
and faster, Blake got back to the house way ahead of his little sister. Eyes alight with wonder, so excited that he was up on the balls
of his feet, Blake stood there in the kitchen and tried to describe
to us what he and Vivienne had just seen. "Mama, Mama, we saw
some, we saw some . . ." He clearly had a deep desire to communicate and share what he saw, but the words simply weren't coming. When Vivienne came racing in behind him a minute later, it
was a whole other story. They'd had the same experience, seen
the same details, and had the same feelings, but Vivienne could
put it in words. A lot of words. And quickly.

"Mommy, Mommy," she said, words pouring out of her excit-
edly, "we saw a whole family of baby ducks, they were really cute,
there were two boys and three girls, they were red and black, except for the mommy duck, who was mostly black and white
and . . ." Vivienne went on and on in tons of detail. Unheard and
upstaged, Blake knocked a magazine off the kitchen counter and
stormed off to his room with tears in his eyes.

Blake is a smart kid. His ability to notice details has always
been incredible. The things he observed and picked up on visually were remarkable for a kid his age. Even as a little guy, he
identified and mimicked animals better than any kid I'd ever
seen. If a topic really interested him and he had a chance to find
the words or could express himself through gestures, acting out,
or imitations, what he sought to communicate was vivid and real.
When he was three, I showed him a picture that accompanied a
newspaper item about an escaped mountain lion. He pointed at
the photo and said, "No. It puma."

"But the article says it's a mountain lion, Blakey," I explained. "No. It puma." He was positive.

Finally I took a closer look. The photo caption read in tiny letters, "Pictured: North American puma." He hadn't read it—he just knew it. A three-by-five black-and-white photo in *USA Today* and he still recognized the difference between a mountain lion and a puma. As long as it was something visual rather than something said or read, he had the opportunity to link a word with a picture, and he was engrossed in the topic at hand, Blake didn't miss a trick. Show him something, point to something, act out something, and he was up to speed. Talking and listening were, unfortunately, another story. He was so smart, yet at school his teachers said he hardly participated. The good news was that he had no temper issues at school. The bad news was that his teachers said he was barely contributing in class.

After talking to Blake's teachers and his speech therapist, we had Blake tested again by an educational evaluator to see whether there was something developmentally wrong with him. This time the results that came back were all over the map. Blakey tested below average for his age on some skills and at an extremely high level for others.

At Blake's speech pathologist's suggestion we went to a speech-language clinic and had him tested by an audiologist for something called auditory processing disorder (APD). The testing confirmed that Blake had this very issue. We were made to understand that this is not at all a rare disorder, but we hadn't heard of it before and we hardly knew what to do with the diagnosis now that we finally had it; we didn't have a clue how to help our son.

From our perspective, our son Blake wasn't a diagnosis or a label—a student who had learning difficulties, a child with APD. He was a human being, a complex and beautiful little guy with a family role to fulfill, schoolwork to do, a growing social world to explore, and a life of potential opportunities, triumphs, tragedies,

mistakes, and successes ahead of him. He needed a way to connect to his family, his teachers, his friends, and the rest of the
world around him to his best advantage. Blake needed a break.
We all did. It just seemed like there was a puzzle to be solved
where Blake was concerned. We had to find someone to help us
acquire the missing pieces, fit them together, and figure it all out.

Then we met Lois Heymann.

On recommendation from Blake's school, Lois came out to
the house and met with us and with Blake. Lois is a speech-
language pathologist who works with children, families, and educators to help kids who are struggling with hearing, listening,
and using language. Her expertise was different from that of the
speech therapist we had seen. Lois wasn't just interested in
Blake's speech output—how he formed and said words. She is a
specialist trained to examine and explore the underlying issues
contributing to Blake's inability to communicate effectively. It
was her job to solve the puzzle. Lois looked at the clinic's test results and then sat down with Blake. She gently asked him questions, patiently checked his answers, and noted what was and
wasn't happening as Blake tried to communicate. She confirmed
that Blake had an APD and explained to Kelli and me that
though Blake could hear just fine for a kid his age—he didn't
have hearing loss or anything physically wrong with his hearing—the parts of Blake's brain in charge of turning sounds into
words and words into language hadn't developed as well as they
should have. What Blake heard wasn't getting processed and
translated the way it should. His acting out at home and nonpar-
ticipation at school were symptoms of his APD. In simple terms,
Blake hadn't learned how to listen. This, Lois explained, was
something different from not paying attention. In fact, Blake was
paying a whole lot of attention, but his brain wasn't creating for
him a deeper understanding of what he was hearing—something
most children do naturally.

Lois explained that every loud environment we took Blake into made it virtually impossible for him to communicate. The noises in the mall and the barbershop had robbed Blake of his ability to focus on what he was being asked, and he hadn't had the extra time he needed to figure out what he was being told and then decide what to say back. The deficiencies in Blake's ability to listen to and comprehend language had held back his vocabulary and speaking skills, Lois said. Even though he'd seen the family of ducks just as clearly and in as much detail as his little sister and was just as excited and eager to tell me about it, he didn't have the words and the word order available to describe what he saw and how he felt. In a calmer, less competitive setting, such as studying the photo of the puma in the newspaper with me, however, he could articulate a great deal. Blake's auditory processing disorder made it hard for him to learn, store, recall, choose, order, and speak words as quickly and naturally as Vivienne.

Lois didn't just explain the puzzle; she had a plan. Her therapy technique is about integrating the exercises that could help Blake as seamlessly as possible into our larger lives, about integrating his needs with our lifestyle. Under her guidance we looked at ways to make our home environment as listening-friendly as possible. We stopped playing loud music, used felt sound dampers under our furniture, and cut down on the size and number of social gatherings we'd have if they were likely to be noisy and chaotic. Lois sat down with Parker, Chelsea, and Vivienne and shared ideas that would help them to better understand what Blake was trying to communicate. She wanted to make sure that we were all by Blake's side as he got back on the road to realizing his true potential. Together, Lois, Kelli, and I met with Blake's school administrators to find ways to make his class environment better suited to focusing on the teacher's voice and the sound of the lesson at hand, not classroom noises and distractions.

Best of all, though, Lois worked directly with us and Blake. In twice-weekly sessions Lois helped us to help Blake build the listening and learning foundation that his APD had kept him from assembling in the first place. Through reading time, rhyming games, language play, and combining sounds with movements and physical touch, Lois began to unlock Blake's language abilities and helped him learn to listen. At first we watched in amazement—it was like she had the code book and was helping us decipher Blake's issues at last. Then we started working and playing with Blake ourselves—reading and talking to him, asking and answering his questions, letting him know what he needed to do, and finally better understanding what he needed from us. In less than a year, Lois and her plan completely transformed our lives.

It wasn't easy. It still isn't sometimes. Working and living with a child with APD takes discipline, and it takes patience. A lot. Progress can be extremely slow. Children with an APD usually have gone for way too long without a lot of the vocabulary and input the rest of us take for granted. The opportunity for a misunderstanding is always around the corner. Without a complete picture of words, gestures, expressions, tones, and meanings working together, kids with APD struggle with humor, puns, and metaphors. Blake doesn't forget anything, but because of his APD he's missed out on a lot. He sometimes still has trouble with figurative talk and off-the-wall humor. I tend to talk in metaphors, so I've had to try not to do that with him, and that's taken some getting used to!

But slow as it has been, the progress we've made has been remarkable, and it's continuing. Lois's supply of listening and learning techniques and strategies, games, activities, and ways to make everyday experiences into listening interactions seems unlimited. After months and months of reading, rhyming, game playing, and changing our style of interacting, all with Blake's auditory processing disorder in mind, the happy, smiling Blake began to visit. Within a year or two he was back to stay. By working with Lois and using her plan, we've helped a new Blake emerge. Now we don't just read to him—he reads to us. The content and easygoing person he appeared to be as an infant has returned.

I watched Lois Heymann lead my child from a world of total confusion, disappointment, and narrow options to one of understanding, enthusiasm, and sky's-the-limit opportunity. Along the way I discovered that listening is the most essential skill our children use to learn, make meaningful personal connections, and live and grow happily. I also learned that listening skills need to be nurtured by all parents. Lois's ideas, information, and exercises collected in *The Sound of Hope* will be a godsend for the family of any child struggling with APD or other listening and learning problems. Having Lois come into our lives certainly was a turning point for my family. But for any mother, father, teacher, or caregiver with a stake in a child's ability to listen, think, experience, and grow, the information in this book will be just as indispensable. Kids learn by listening, and *The Sound of Hope* gives both parents and children the keys to open the door on a big, beautiful world of possibility.

—Rosie O'Donnell

INTRODUCTION

The act of listening—using our ears and our mind together to interpret and experience sound and language in the fullest possible way—is one of life's great pleasures. The beauty of a musical melody, the reassuring sound of a loved one's voice, and the sheer joy of understanding and appreciating what's being done and said around us are simply irreplaceable. But the act of listening is also a vital skill, one that needs to be learned and honed over time.

The simple truth is that listening is the key that unlocks a child's ability to learn. Educators estimate that children spend 70 percent of their day listening, yet there are no classes that teach students this essential skill. Children need years of practice to develop the ability to listen to instructions, absorb and make sense of spoken and heard information, and follow directions. They're expected to enter kindergarten already able to use these skills. That means it's up to parents to teach their children how to be good lis-

teners and effective communicators at home and prepare them
for the educational and social challenges they'll face in school.

Today's parents are hard at work raising the first generations
to grow up in the digital age. Their challenge is to balance the benefits that technology can offer with the critical gift of learning
through listening and human interaction. The Internet, digital
television, handheld music players and video games, cell phones,
and everything else being cooked up in Silicon Valley bombard
you and your kids with sounds, words, images, and information at
a rate no other generation has ever had to navigate. While it's great
to have so many communication and entertainment tools at our
fingertips, that new flood tide of words, images, and sounds can be
so relentless that you can scarcely make sense of it—and if you're
struggling, imagine what your children are grappling with.

When children are cocooned inside the digital world—surfing the Internet, watching TV, or playing video games—the very
necessary interaction with the real world of voices and ideas is the
first thing to go. Childhood is a time when physical, emotional,
and intellectual development should weave together harmoniously. Just as your child's physical coordination and strength
grow through repetition and experience, your child's listening
ability increases according to his or her own natural ability and
feeling for language, words, and rhythm. In the rush to give our
children every advantage, we may have overlooked those basic
auditory needs. The simple one-on-one games that parents and
children have shared for generations are still the best way to enhance your child's ability to listen and learn. Singing, rhyming,
playing, and reading with our children provide a necessary and
irreplaceable foundation for learning.

The challenge to learn through the skill of listening is even
greater for children who are either born with or develop a dis-
connect between their ears' ability to hear and their brain's ability
to make sense and use out of the sound information that their ears

pass on. Children with what's become known as (central) auditory processing disorders (CAPD or more commonly APD) can hear, but for a variety of reasons they can't make ear and mind consistently work together to listen effectively. As many as three in every hundred children suffer from an APD that affects the brain's ability to recognize and interpret speech and language sounds accurately. For these children, every experience with language—the words and instructions their parents and teachers say to them, the jokes they share and the games they play with their friends and classmates—carries a burden of confusion and frustration.

Children with an APD encounter nearly insurmountable obstacles to understanding, learning, and enjoying themselves each and every day. Inability or difficulty transforming passive hearing into active listening makes academics challenging to master and many social situations emotionally painful and difficult to endure. Left unidentified (through screening), undiagnosed (through evaluation), and untreated (through coordinated therapy and intervention), an auditory processing disorder can hold an otherwise bright and willing child back for life.

But where there are words there is hope. The sound of hope is the sound of engaged and loving parents and other family members along with committed and concerned teachers and caregivers using the ideas, strategies, games, songs, and rhymes in this book to awaken and nurture the ability to listen and communicate in a growing child, whether listening comes easily and naturally or not. The same extra loving attention and carefully planned activities and exercises that made a difference for Rosie O'Donnell's family can help any family cope with and triumph over the very real and often sadly misunderstood struggle to listen effectively that burdens children with APD and threatens any child growing up in the information age.

Diagnosing an APD in a young child is difficult. The true nature and magnitude of an individual auditory processing disorder can't really be gauged until your child is school age. That's why this book has been created to help parents who suspect their child may be struggling with listening skills or who want to give their daughter or son an extra boost and attention in that area. I've spent thirty years working as a speech-language pathologist— a specialist who deals with hearing, listening, and language problems and therapies. In that time I've enjoyed the privilege of getting to know and to help hundreds of children who need extra assistance in listening, learning, and communicating using words, sounds, and voices. It's also been my pleasure to meet and work with parents such as Rosie who are looking for ways to best meet their child's needs and to integrate their child's therapy into their family's lives. My job requires that I listen, too. What I've heard from children and parents has helped me to appreciate what parents want and children need the most—to share a deep sense of connection and a powerful sense of purpose that ultimately becomes a joyful and playful process.

If you have children, then you know that there's no set formula for raising them. Every day, week, month, and year in a child's growth and life brings its own challenges. The strategies, ideas, and activities I describe can be made to fit into you and your child's unique and individual lives. You can make the games, rhymes, and books you share more or less challenging, depending on your child's specific age and needs. Any child from infancy to age eight can benefit from the parenting ideas I've created, collected, and arranged in *The Sound of Hope*.

Each chapter of *The Sound of Hope* focuses on a particular aspect of your child's development and offers tested, clear, and simple ways for you and your child to enhance and improve that development. Just as I do with my clients, I will help you teach your child to enhance, fully utilize, and enjoy his or her natural abilities as a listener, learner, and communicator. We'll travel layer by layer through your child's development while recognizing that growth is always overlapping and that you can pick and choose exercises and games from any point and mix and match them along the way. I'll also help you to become aware of roadblocks and obstacles that I've helped clients to overcome in one-on-one sessions. In the final chapter I'll share some ideas and information about getting additional help and finding a speech-language pathologist, audiologist, or other professional in your area.

The techniques you'll learn have already enabled hundreds of parents to balance the demands of their busy lives with the dreams they have for their families. I know that they will work for you as well. These exercises are important—and they're fun, too. Having fun talking, reading, laughing, singing, and rhyming together optimizes the teaching time that the two of you will spend together, helps to fit those lessons into the framework of your busy lives, means that they can be adjusted in length and frequency to fit any schedule, and, most of all, offers great ways for you and your child to enjoy each other's company. It only takes a little preparation and a few minutes each day to turn everyday activities you already share with your child into powerful listening lessons and priceless quality time.

The Sound of Hope can change the way you think about listening. It offers a new way of looking at childhood development by focusing on the importance of listening as a cornerstone of social and academic success. One of the most satisfying and rewarding experiences in life is to learn something new. *The Sound of Hope* is a guide to giving your child as many of these moments as possible.

PART ONE

RECOGNIZING AND UNDERSTANDING APD

ONE

When Hearing Isn't Listening: The ABCs of APD

M argaret's beautiful baby boy Billy Ray was six months old when she began to sense that something wasn't right. Why didn't Billy Ray look at her, even when Margaret took him in her arms and murmured his name? Margaret had a powerful sense that the sounds her little boy made, so different in pitch and tone from her first child's coos and giggles, were just, well, wrong. And Margaret rarely had any sense that her son was making his baby sounds in response to the things his mom said or did.

Her doctor assured her there was nothing to worry about. "Boys start to talk later than girls," he explained. "Besides, Billy Ray is the second child in the family. His need to communicate with you is not as great." *Well, he's the doctor,* Margaret thought. Yet in her heart, she just couldn't accept these reasonable-sounding explanations. Margaret felt deep down that Billy Ray should be responding more to her and her husband's voices and the sounds and noises in their home. Based on her experience with her first child, she sensed that the pre-speech vocalizations

Billy Ray made should be different from what they were. Reaching for a box of rice one afternoon at home, Margaret impulsively rattled it behind Billy Ray's head. When he again failed to react, Margaret knew what she had to do. The following day, she had Billy Ray's hearing checked, fully expecting that her child had a hearing impairment.

The results came back normal.

Undeterred, Margaret arranged for consultations with two separate pediatric neurologists. After a battery of tests and examinations with Billy Ray and a lengthy interview with Margaret, both doctors concluded that Billy Ray had pervasive developmental disorder (PDD). Margaret had never heard of PDD, a condition involving developmental delays of socialization and communication skills. She tried to be as upbeat as possible as each neurologist explained what PDD was and described a therapeutic preschool and the necessary therapy that would accommodate Billy Ray's special needs. Margaret was grateful for the diagnosis—having one gave her something new to focus her efforts on—but worried that the doctors were sentencing her beautiful little boy to a life of isolation. Nevertheless, Margaret did the research, fought with her insurance company, and adjusted her family's budget so that Billy Ray could attend the school and receive the therapy that both doctors recommended.

But by age two Billy Ray was still uncommunicative. Worse, as he grew from infant to toddler, Billy Ray's inability to listen began to be an educational and social ball and chain for him. Frustrated by an invisible wall that complicated and confused nearly everything he was asked to do, Billy Ray cried and acted out a lot. Unable to state his own needs or understand what other boys and girls asked for, he pushed and grabbed for toys, upsetting his peers and testing his teachers' patience. As his mother looked on helplessly, Billy Ray increasingly retreated into a world of his own. Instead of each new day offering a chance to grow, develop, and interact more meaningfully and happily with the world around him, Margaret, Billy Ray, and their family faced a daily struggle simply to cope.

Margaret could see how much it hurt and confused Billy Ray when he misunderstood and was in turn misunderstood, but she was at a loss as to how best to help her son. It felt as if Billy Ray was on the other side of a door, knocking for her to unlock it, and Margaret simply didn't have the key. Increasingly Margaret worried that if she couldn't find a way to open the door and lead Billy Ray out into the full, rich world of experience, her little boy would never be able to play and connect with his sister, make friends in school, fall in love, go to college, or live on his own. Margaret redoubled the hunt for the key. There must be something she'd missed, someone she hadn't consulted. She made calls, quizzed other parents, scanned parenting websites and chat boards, and read and reread everything she could find about Billy Ray's diagnosed disorder, PDD.

Along the way she happened upon a website that described yet another three-letter syndrome. When she read the symptoms of APD or auditory processing disorder, she could scarcely believe it. Here was the exact list of what Billy Ray was going through. Children with APD:

- Have trouble listening and hearing, especially in noisy environments
- Struggle to distinguish between similar-sounding words and sounds
- Don't follow directions well
- Frequently ask for clarification and to have words repeated
- Do poorly in reading and reading comprehension, spelling, and other classes where verbal directions are key
- Fare better in independent activities and classes where listening isn't a central requirement

One other item made her sit bolt upright:

- Are often misdiagnosed with other disorders such as ADD (attention deficit disorder), ADHD (attention deficit hyperactivity disorder), and pervasive developmental delay (PDD)

Intrigued—and hopeful that perhaps there would be more that she could do for Billy Ray if *this* was his true problem—Margaret started to look further and asked more questions of the growing list of specialists she'd already consulted. She felt she was on the path to discovering how to unlock the proverbial door for her son.

Margaret is certainly not alone in her search to help unlock the door to healthy development for her son. If you're reading this book, you likely suspect that your own child has one of these three-letter syndromes, or you already have a suggested diagnosis in hand and are trying to digest as much information as possible going forward.

Generally speaking, *auditory processing disorder* is a term for a group of conditions in which the parts of a child's brain tasked with turning sound into language and hearing into listening don't do their jobs right. How this issue develops and at what age it most often does so is little understood—we'll discuss this more below—but it is estimated that between 1.5 million and 2.5 million children a year are diagnosed with this disorder. Because auditory pathways leading from the ear into the brain and the auditory processing centers within the brain itself are continuously developing throughout infancy and early childhood, it's not possible to screen for and definitively establish the presence of an APD in a child until she or he is six or seven years old. A specific diagnosis detailing the magnitude of the APD as well as any related or concurrent problems such as ADD or ADHD and the right course of therapy and treatment cannot in turn be made until the child is seven or eight. But there are clearly many, many more younger children dealing with these listening difficulties. We think some children are even born with this issue. Unfortunately, because the development of auditory processing skills is linked with a growing child's use of language and increasingly complex communications and social interactions and cannot be accurately measured until those skills develop, parents have to go without formal diagnosis and intervention for too long. The ideas in this book will help you understand what's at stake in your child's listening development and in turn help your child from the moment you begin to suspect that there may be a problem. You don't need to wait for a formal diagnosis to begin to help.

THE ABCS OF APD

In broad strokes, it's easiest to understand hearing—the process of experiencing sound—as a two-stage phenomenon. First, sound vibrations are collected by the outer ear, funneled to the inner ear, where they become physical vibrations, and then sent on to the cochlea, where they are transformed into electrical impulses. Then these impulses travel along the eighth cranial nerve into the brain.

As the electrical impulses enter and go deeper into the brain, they pass through a series of relay stations in which the auditory information they carry is analyzed for timing (duration), intensity (volume), and frequency (pitch). The sound signals from each ear also get switched over like railcars changing tracks and are rerouted to the opposite side of the brain. Sound received in the right ear is sent to the left auditory cortex, while sound from the left ear goes to the right auditory cortex. The auditory cortex is a specialized area within the cerebral cortex that organizes, analyzes, and transforms sound information into the sensations and reactions that we recognize as language and speech. For most people the left cortex does the lion's share of the work.

Once inside these brain centers, sound impulses are put

A couple of years ago, Kelli took Blake and his younger sister, Vivienne, to see Legally Blonde *on Broadway. Everyone loved the play so much that when they got home they were still talking about it. Vivienne was dying to tell me that the lead character in the show had the same first name as her. This was news to Blake. He stated defiantly and absolutely that his sister and the girl in the play didn't have the same name at all. Vivi quickly countered, in her typical rapid-fire delivery, "Yes, we do too have the same name, Blake. My name is Vivienne and the girl in the play's name is Viviane. She has blond hair and I have blond hair, and . . ." We all nodded and agreed. I checked the* Playbill. *Sure enough, the title character's name was Viviane. Blake took the difference in opinion personally, kicked the leg of a table, yelled "No," and ran up the stairs to his bedroom, slamming the door behind him. Kelli and I looked at each other and sighed. I waited a few minutes to give Blake a chance to settle down before I walked upstairs, knocked on his door, and went in to talk to him about what had just happened. "Blake," I asked him, "what was the girl's name in the play?" "Bibienne," he answered. He heard it differently than his sister and everyone else in the theater. If he'd been actively listening, he might have realized that what he heard didn't make sense the way he heard it. The truth is, no one really listens all the time and no two people listen or speak exactly the same way. It's easy to take for granted that what one kid hears will be the same that another hears. But Blake hears differently than Vivienne and he speaks differently than she does. In any family a little extra attention to exactly who's getting what out of what's being said can really pay off.*

—ROSIE

through a highly sophisticated and detailed battery of analyses and examinations contoured by memory, instinct, thought, and various voluntary and involuntary reactions into the sensation we experience as hearing. It's a complex process—one that simultaneously incorporates multiple locations of brain geography, a system of feedback to the cochlea to help narrow the focus of hearing, and a myriad of other analyses, impulses, gateways, functions, and processes. All this happens in a fraction of a second.

Most people recognize that birth defects, infections, blockages, eardrum punctures, tinnitus from loud noises, and various other things can adversely affect the middle and inner ear, important parts of the hearing equation. But a lot can also go wrong during a sound's journey along the eighth cranial nerve through the relay stations and inside the auditory cortex. APD is a condition that affects that interior trip to the auditory cortex and the processing stage that transforms hearing into listening within the cortex itself.

THE DEVELOPMENTAL LADDER

Since we don't yet know what causes APD and can't predict at what age it may develop, it's important to understand the typical developmental milestones common to most young children. These developmental milestones are a loose guide. They can help you to zero in on your child's listening development. If your child's listening and speaking skills don't come anywhere near the trajectory I describe, APD may be the problem. Keep in mind that the ideas, observations, and indications that follow are not one-size-fits-all. A child's journey to developmental maturity is a ladder of many rungs. Your son or daughter can pause on one rung longer than another child the same age, skip one, or even go back a few and still be well within the range of "normal." Always keep in mind that variation and individual timing is the natural order of things when it comes to growing children.

Birth to Three Months

- ✓ Newborns listen to sounds that are close to them.
- ✓ Unexpected or loud sounds may startle them or make them cry.
- ✓ New and interesting sounds may calm them or cause them to stop movement and "listen" or attend. Recognizing attention in a newborn can be tricky at first. Sometimes it's visible only in an interruption of sucking on a pacifier or a bottle.
- ✓ The baby begins to localize and turn in the direction of a sound source.
- ✓ A familiar voice gets greeted with a familiar expression, sound, or gesture.
- ✓ The baby responds to soft, comforting tones.

In the first ninety days of life, a newborn infant is fully occupied by the basic needs for comfort, food, rest, hygiene, and love. During these first beautiful months your baby spends most of his or her day sleeping and being kept clean, fed, and adored. At the same time that your baby begins to develop a sense of touch she also begins to respond to the trust and warmth she soaks up from the people who care for her. By the third month your baby begins to grasp and hold things such as rattles and stuffed animals, and fully expects that her comfort and contact needs will be met.

Initially your baby communicates by crying. You and the other adults around her begin to read her signals and recognize that the specific cry for being hungry is different from the cry for being wet. Soon she will start making other sounds and playing with her growing ability to vocalize; she will repeat sounds that get your attention and approval.

Three to Six Months

✓ Sounds begin to have meaning.
✓ A child begins to respond to "no."
✓ The baby recognizes changes in a voice's loudness and pitch.
✓ He or she starts to associate word meaning with sound.
✓ The baby listens to his or her own voice.
✓ Rhythm and music draw their own reaction.
✓ The baby shows an interest in toys that pair sound with movement, such as rattles, musical mobiles, or anything else designed to make noise when it moves or is moved.
✓ The baby demonstrates increased attention to more varied environmental sounds, such as a vacuum cleaner, a fan, or a door slamming in another room.

At the ninety-day mark, your baby is now ready to play. She is awake for longer periods of time, is more physically active and clearly enjoys interacting with you. She can now grasp objects and bring them to her mouth for more sensory exploration. If your play involves language, your baby is ready to experience that, too. At this age a child can create vowel-like ("a," "e," "o") and consonant-like ("p," "b," "m") sounds.

Six to Twelve Months

✓ The child begins to listen and pay attention when spoken to.
✓ He or she responds to his or her name by turning.
✓ He or she is able to focus on listening for longer periods of time.
✓ The baby begins to like and play games that pair voice with movements.

✓ Familiar words (names of daily used objects and frequently seen people) are recognized in familiar contexts.
✓ The baby responds to familiar requests, such as waving
bye-bye or being asked to give something to the parent.
✓ The child recognizes sounds paired with objects, such as an
animal sound with the appropriate animal.

Your baby is awake even more and therefore more available to
play. At six to twelve months a baby loves to look at books and pictures with you and is becoming much more physically active. She's
developing a longer attention span, sitting by herself, crawling,
pulling herself up to standing, and possibly even taking her first
steps. She shows off her developing fine motor skills while playing
with blocks and stacking rings. As the twelve-month mark approaches, she clearly understands more about the world around her.

One to Two Years

✓ The child begins to show specific comprehension of words.
✓ He or she can point out and identify pictures and objects by
their names.
✓ He or she can also point to simple body parts on themselves
and others.
✓ The child will now imitate words he or she hears.
✓ The child can follow one-step commands or questions such
as "Throw the ball" or "Where's the kitty?"
✓ He or she likes listening to simple stories.
✓ The child loves to listen to songs and rhymes and can incor-
porate body and hand movements to go with some of them.

During this time your baby's speech makes a big leap forward.
Over the course of year one to two, most children go from babbling
to creating nonsense words to learning and using real words and fi-

nally to using real words in two-word combinations. Increasingly your child enjoys playing with things that represent actual objects, such as using a block as a truck. She also explores her environment, learning how to walk and even how to climb stairs and using fine motor skills to manipulate simple one-piece puzzles.

Two to Three Years

✓ The child's understanding broadens to include following two-step commands such as "Pick up your crayons and put them in the box."

✓ He or she attaches meanings and activities to environmental sounds, such as attempting to answer a ringing phone or running to the door at the sound of a doorbell.

✓ The child begins to understand concepts and their opposites, including hot/cold, up/down, and stop/go.

During this year your child starts using sentences and conversation begins. She's walking, maybe riding a tricycle, and using increasingly complicated toys, such as interlocking blocks, to build and play.

Three to Four Years

✓ The child can hear and understand at increasing distances from the source of a sound.

✓ He or she understands questions such as "who," "what," and "where."

✓ Social interactions with other children become more important.

✓ The child listens to longer stories.

✓ Attention span increases at this age.

✓ The child can now link two separate pieces of information into one.

A three-to-four-year-old is a very busy little person. Children of this age get involved with other children more as play becomes increasingly interactive, especially outside at the playground. They also like "helping" around the house. Because she is around other children more, your child will hear and say things she's never heard or said before and begin to tell stories. Her fine motor skill development has progressed, so she can play games with smaller pieces. Simple board games and drawing and coloring become favorite activities.

Four to Five Years

- ✓ Enjoyment and understanding of stories deepen. The child is now able to answer questions about the stories and shows increasing comprehension.
- ✓ He or she is able to take turns in a conversation by understanding and listening for the cues that indicate turn taking.
- ✓ The child understands longer and more complex sentences.
- ✓ He or she retells longer stories with more details.

By this age a child's language and narrative skills have progressed and she's able to grasp a pencil and begin to write. She's also becoming more independent and dressing herself. Four- and five-year-olds love ball games and start learning and playing games that have rules.

THE CAUSES OF APD

The root cause of a condition that plagues so many perfectly intelligent children with normal hearing in the United States alone is still under study and discussion. Clinical observation hasn't offered up a single genetic, environmental, physical, or developmental smoking gun behind APD. But as doctors, scientists, and therapists work to unlock its secrets and treat its symptoms, several general factors associated with auditory processing disorder have drawn increasing scrutiny.

CHILDREN ARE MORE AT RISK FOR APD:

- After complicated births. Newborns who endure physically traumatic arrivals appear more likely to develop an auditory processing disorder.
- After premature births. Preemies are sometimes born with an immature or weakened sensory system, affecting their ability to effectively process sound.
- In the aftermath of chronic middle ear infections (otitis media).
- In boys more than girls. In my practice I see boys and girls with APD or APD symptoms in about equal numbers, but some sources observe that two-thirds of children with APD are male.
- In children that have been neglected or isolated after birth.

From day one a healthy child with undamaged hearing needs to hear sounds that will encourage his or her brain to install and streamline the pathways and connections that make speech and language possible. A household or living situation where a newborn is exposed to manageable amounts of quality language and sound is simply vital to developing the skill of listening. If a child arrives in the world and is placed in an environment that doesn't address this need, his auditory processing skills may not develop the way they should. APD is often seen in children who have been neglected at birth. While many adopted children receive the necessary auditory developmental boost from attentive caregivers and foster parents, some children are born into situations where they had to subsist on the bare minimum necessary to survive, let alone develop, learn, and grow. The good news is that with interventions such as the ones offered later in this book, parents and caregivers can begin to make up for these early deficits and foster the neural connections that were not nurtured early in a child's life.

WHAT IT'S LIKE TO HAVE APD

At the simplest level, a child with APD struggles with using sound to listen. This primary difficulty becomes the root cause of a wide variety of developmental, educational, and behavioral symptoms. Over time APD-related symptoms can worsen, combine, and increase in number as the condition goes undiagnosed and the child goes untreated.

AT HOME AND AT PLAY FROM INFANCY TO PRESCHOOL:

- The child may not respond appropriately or consistently to what's been said or heard—even calling his name can cause different reactions at different times.
- The child can't pinpoint where a sound is coming from.
- When spoken to or expected to interact or play in a situation that relies on talk and sound without anything visual to back it up, the child gets easily distracted or quickly bored.
- Loud noises and noisy environments may upset, anger, or frighten the child, while quiet rooms, places, and activities may calm and reassure him.
- The beginning of a poor memory for words and numbers shows up. Simple vocabulary such as the ABCs, days of the week, names of everyday objects, and names of familiar

people goes unlearned. Similar-sounding words become difficult to distinguish from each other and comprehend separately.

Successfully processing sounds and words is a constantly growing skill set the child takes to his first school experience. A child with APD faces increasing struggles in school, at home, and in the world outside.

IN PRESCHOOL:

- A child with APD has a hard time following directions, especially when the directions are not part of a familiar routine and the child doesn't have any visual cues such as pictures or familiar gestures from teachers to go with them.
- Many directions and questions posed by adults get a "Huh?" or "What?" and a baffled expression from the child.
- Forming sentences and building vocabulary comes more slowly and with a lot more difficulty than for the other boys and girls in class.
- The APD preschooler leaves sounds and syllables out of words or substitutes sounds that make what he or she says difficult for teachers and classmates to follow.
- The background noise of a busy preschool environment poses an increasing challenge to a child with APD. Loud situations become an irresistible distraction or a source of emotional upset. A conventionally noisy environment can prevent him or her from understanding what's being explained, asked, or said.
- The songs and rhymes that other children learn together and on their own are very hard for the child with APD to get the hang of. Riddles and jokes may make no sense to the child at all.

Working with Andy, a seven-year-old child with APD, one day, I suggested that we write a story together.

"What will we write it in?" Andy asked me.

"In your composition book," I replied, making sure to look right at him and point to the notebook in my hand.

"What's a *competition* book?" Andy asked. Andy was very smart and very sensitive, and I could tell he was already frustrated that my answer to his question made no sense. Andy hadn't heard all the sounds of the words I spoke, and substituted a word he already knew for the one that I actually said. For a girl or boy who doesn't have APD, this is a simple mistake in conversation. But for a boy like Andy, this single mismatch of words was one of dozens of mistakes, misunderstandings, and miscommunications he'd endured so far that day. The child with APD is crushed under the weight of all these piled-up misunderstandings and the embarrassment and frustration that come with using the wrong word and not getting the gist of a conversation or instruction. With other children his age, it's even worse. The eye rolling, tactless comments, and impatience these little mistakes provoke all day long from Andy's peers make it hard for an otherwise perfectly intelligent and sweet little boy to keep up self-esteem, find his way among his classmates, and make friends.

- The child increasingly relies on pictures, illustrations, gestures, and other visual information.
- Social communication and the beginnings of conversation with other girls and boys his or her age are full of misunderstandings and often lead to hurt feelings and fights.
- Complex language such as metaphors ("You little piggies

will need to clean up this mess before snack time," "Aren't you a busy bee?") and figurative verbal examples ("We have enough food here to feed an army!" "Why, you're covered with dirt from head to toe!") are simply baffling to a child with APD.

INTO KINDERGARTEN AND FIRST GRADE, THESE PROBLEMS JUST GET WORSE

- Distraction and inattention become a constant problem for the kindergarten and primary school student with APD.
- Language development—growing vocabulary, grammar skills, sentence structure, and ability to listen—don't progress on schedule. Spelling and reading skills come slowly or not at all.
- Multistep directions are endlessly challenging.
- The constant "Huh?" and "What?" of preschool evolves into a frustrated reliance on "I don't know" and "I don't understand" in many verbal activities.
- The child with APD performs well in activities only when sound information is backed up with visuals.
- The slow development, inarticulateness, and inattentiveness of an APD first grader can mimic the symptoms of ADD and/or hearing loss.
- Poorly evolving social communication skills with other boys and girls and with teachers add to a child with APD's increasing isolation and unhappiness.
- Organizational skills don't develop in line with other children's.
- The kindergartner or primary school student with APD opts out of class discussions or appears lost and gives answers that are not on the topic at hand.

TWO

Confusing APD with Other Three-Letter Syndromes

APD symptoms and treatments cover several different specific listening difficulties and have a number of different possible causes. While difficulties with any of the situations and developmental markers I've listed for various ages can mean your child has an APD, too often children with a bona fide auditory processing disorder are misdiagnosed with another condition that has a three-letter acronym. Indeed, since a diagnosis of APD is often made once other problems have been ruled out, it's helpful to think of APD in terms of what it is *not*.

APD IS NOT HEARING LOSS

Hearing loss is the result of problems in the middle ear or inner ear. Anything that goes wrong along the chain of membranes, bones, and organs that make up the middle and inner ear can cause hearing loss. Fluid buildup, infection, scarring or blockage in the middle ear, birth defects affecting the middle or inner ear's anatomy, damage to the hairs within the cochlea—these are all conditions that can cause a temporary or permanent loss of hearing. Some of these conditions can be screened and initially diagnosed by a speech pathologist, a pediatrician or an otolaryngologist (what used to be called an ear-nose-throat doctor). The type and severity of the hearing loss needs to be gauged by an audiologist. Depending on how severe the hearing loss is and what caused it, doctors, along with an audiologist and a speech-language pathologist, can present parents with options so that they can decide what course to take. Different types and severities of hearing loss respond to different treatments. Hearing aids, prescriptions, therapy sessions, corrective surgery, and surgical implants can each be used to deal with different kinds of hearing loss.

APD is a condition with root causes inside the brain's central auditory nervous system itself, not the middle or inner ear. A child with APD is physically equipped and capable of hearing, but the brain processing that turns hearing into listening just isn't doing its job properly. To diagnose auditory processing disorder an audiologist first has to rule out hearing loss. Once a child has been tested and found to have the physical ability to receive sounds through hearing, the audiologist can test for APD, diagnose the areas of auditory weakness, and recommend the right course of therapeutic action for the APD-affected child.

APD IS NOT ADD, ADHD, OR PDD

Imagine being a young child on a trip to the neighborhood grocery store. The aisles are crowded with customers talking to each other, using cell phones, picking products off the shelves. Freezer doors sigh open and thump closed. Metal shopping carts rattle by. Checkout stations bleep and blip as products are scanned; registers snap open and shut. Announcements and ambient music are piped in through speakers. In the midst of this deep, dense forest of sound your mother says, "We need some milk. Can you get one of the big containers with the blue cap?"

Your ears pick up the ocean of sound waves that you're swimming in and the sounds of the words your mother just said, but your brain is only partially sorting out the auditory information your ears send to it. What you actually hear is: "_____ need _____ milk. Can you _____ one _____ the _____ containers _____ the _____ cap?"

Eager to please your mom, you rush to the dairy case and grab a quart of milk.

"Is that a big container?" she asks.

You look at the small bottle in your hands and shake your head.

"Does it have a blue cap?"

You don't hear what she says at first. She repeats it, and you shake your head again and start to fidget as you see that familiar expression on her face.

"Why can't you *listen*?" she cries.

Even if you only made out part of what she said, your mother's unhappiness and annoyance are clear. A child with an undiagnosed APD is constantly eliciting angry, confused, impatient, disapproving, and upset reactions from immediate family, teachers, and the world at large. Frustrated beyond your ability to cope with an unfair and misunderstood burden, you have a full meltdown in the dairy aisle. It becomes so bad that your mother has to stop shopping and take you out to the car.

Listening is such an essential skill that when a child simply can't do it, it creates a tragic domino effect. As a child grows, the complexity of his interactions with people grows, too. At an age when children are naturally compiling the first few pages of a developing instruction manual for how their world works, APD sees to it that important information is left out. With every un-

> *There are so many different disorders and names for kids' listening and learning problems nowadays that they tend to lump them into one big group. When it's your own kid, sometimes you can't step back and see what's really going on.*
>
> —ROSIE

successful social transaction, incomplete task, and missed point in school, the child with APD is being programmed to fail. APD's toll on listening begins a sequence of falling developmental dominos that can reach into adulthood. Untreated, APD can drastically distort social and educational experiences of every kind. The child retreats into his own head. Disinterest in the surrounding social world, which he is unable to reasonably sort out, coupled with problems communicating and learning, appears to parents, teachers, and doctors alike as an attention problem. To the inexperienced observer, the child's moodiness, tantrums, social isolation, and peer group clumsiness seem like a behavioral problem.

Like a child with ADD, ADHD, or PDD, a child with auditory processing disorder can be:

- Mentally and emotionally exhausted at the end of the day. Struggling to understand at such a young age is a grueling workout.
- Irritable. Feelings of helplessness and an inability to communicate breed anxiety and frustration.
- Low on self-esteem. First and foremost, children blame themselves when things aren't right.
- Negative about school. "It's just too hard" becomes the mantra of a school-age child with APD.
- Seen as immature for her age. Children who are cut off from listening tend to stay put emotionally. A child with

APD will shy away from potentially complex, healthily challenging experiences and encounters. Though he or she is perfectly intelligent, the meaning of jokes, puns, riddles, sarcasm, and other types of wordplay is often lost on a child with APD. Uncomfortable with abstract language and inexperienced in recognizing or detecting how vocal intonation changes the meaning of what is being said, the child has difficulty reading the situation.

These things can all be symptoms of attention and developmental disorders. APD is, however, simply an inability to listen caused by the brain's incomplete or unsuccessful processing of auditory information. A child with APD may have trouble with attention, but it's because she can't listen accurately, not because she can't pay attention. While APD can coexist in a child with ADD, ADHD, or other developmental difficulties, children with APD only are not usually hyperactive. They may engage in impulsive and disruptive behavior like children with those other developmental disorders, but only because of their inability to understand and to be understood. Also, while untreated APD can take a terrible toll in school, it primarily affects the language-oriented parts of learning, unlike ADD. A child with APD can actually do well in math while struggling with speaking, listening, and reading.

APD CANNOT BE TREATED WITH DRUGS OR SURGERY

The symptoms of ADD and the family of attention-based disorders are often successfully treated with prescription drugs. In many cases hearing loss responds well to the recommended treatments, including hearing aids, surgery, and the miraculous evolving technology of cochlear implants. Thus far there is no known prescription or medical procedure that lessens the severity of APD.

Remember Billy Ray and his mother, Margaret? The audiologist that diagnosed Billy Ray referred Margaret to a clinic that specializes in APD. Together the therapists at the clinic, Margaret and her husband, and Billy Ray's teachers began to address the boy's needs—spending patient hours working with him and with each other to see that Billy Ray was given the chance he deserved to learn to listen and become a participating part of the family that loved him and the world around him. It took years of trial and error, many hours of dealing with schools and transforming the home environment, and day after day of reading and playing together, fighting back tears, soothing hurt feelings, and being patient and focused, but Margaret persevered and Billy Ray began to improve. The little boy who was thought to have a developmental disability so severe that it would keep him back in school and social life for years graduated from high school last May and is starting college in the fall.

As difficult as it is to identify the precise nature of the malfunction between hearing and listening that causes an auditory processing disorder, you are not helpless in the face of an APD. You already possess the single most effective tool for dealing with your child's unique situation: a parent's caring, nurturing love. The second essential weapon in the fight against APD is knowledge, and in the next chapter I'll share a very important piece of information every parent should have in place before using and expressing their caring, nurturing love through helping their child cope and grow beyond an APD's limitations. Before we can apply ourselves to undoing and lessening the harm of an APD, we'll need to be clear on the fundamentals of the skill of listening itself.

THREE

The Developmental Elements
of Listening

Before you can fully understand and appreciate your vital role in teaching your child to turn hearing into listening, it helps to have a functional knowledge of just what goes into listening at its most basic. In his book *Auditory Training* Dr. Norman P. Erber, audiologist and consultant in issues of hearing loss, narrowed the skill of listening to a four-part sequence made up of:

1. Detection
2. Discrimination
3. Identification
4. Comprehension

THE FOUR PARTS OF LISTENING

Detection

Detection is the on/off switch of hearing and listening—the move from nothing to something. Imagine that you clap your hands. Your palms come together and produce a chain reaction of sound waves. A child playing nearby in a comparatively quiet sound environment will effectively go from sensing less or no sound to more sound—specifically, that one particularly loud sound of a hand clap. Detecting a sound is the first level of auditory processing within the brain.

Discrimination

Sound is never a specific, single, homogenous thing. Water can take the form of ocean waves, a trickle from a faucet, chunks of ice, scalding steam, slow seepage up from the ground, or a blast from a fire hose. Air can be cold, hot, a gentle breeze, a strong wind, a puff between pursed lips, or a draft under the door. Sound comes to us in just as many intensities and qualities. Once a child has detected a sound, his or her brain must be able to separate that individual sound from whatever other noises—loud, soft, shrill, melodic, rhythmic, monotonous—that may be occurring at the same time. Hearing the hand clap, the child's auditory system transforms the sound into electrical brain impulses and sends it on its way to the auditory cortex of the brain for complete processing. Along the way, that electrical signal is separated from any other auditory signals also going into the brain. Using the brain's ability to discriminate, a baby will distinguish between the specific sound of a clap and, say, the music from a mobile hung above its crib, your voice, the noise of a doorbell ringing, a dog barking, or any other sounds it has experienced thus far in its life.

This ability to discriminate between sounds becomes particularly critical as your child begins to assemble words out of their component sounds. The sounds "buh," "eh," and "duh" may sound similar to your child, but when properly discriminated from one another they form the word "bed."

Identification

Identification involves comparing the sound detected and discriminated from any other sounds the child has previously experienced and has stored in her or his memory. Is it the doorbell? Is it a dog barking? Discrimination says no. Having identified what a sound *is not,* identification goes a step further as the child's brain establishes what the sound *is:* "It's a clap. I have heard this before."

Comprehension

Imagine you are walking past a Broadway theater stage door at the end of a sold-out performance. You hear a distinctive sound (detection) that is different from other sounds you know (discrimination): the sound of clapping (identification). All this happens instantly. But the auditory processing doesn't stop there. Rather than stopping at just mechanically experiencing the sound of clapping, in the final stage of auditory processing, your brain assigns meaning to the sound. As you hear it come out of the stage door, you refine and redefine that clapping as an ovation and experience a mental picture of a very appreciative audience at the end of a show. The same happens to a child hearing a single clap. A baby may be startled or amused by a clap. A toddler may interpret the clap as approval or the start of a song or rhyme. In a preschool classroom it may mean that a teacher is trying to get the children's attention or signaling that an activity is over. As a

During daily routines at home, we try to measure out the directions we give Blake one or two simple steps at a time. When there are multiple tasks to be completed, we take them action by action and allow Blake to complete one or two tasks first before delegating another. We try not to give directions like "After you eat your breakfast, go get dressed, then put your clothes in the laundry basket. Oh, don't forget to brush your teeth and your hair, too." Even though this is a common way to speak, we realize that too many instructions can give Blake too much to work with. It's better for him to take it a step at a time. "It's time to eat your breakfast"; then, once he has eaten, on to the next task or two: "Go get dressed," "Put your dirty clothes in the laundry basket," and so on.

On the other hand, when the family goes out for special occasions, we try to prepare Blake by giving him as many exact details and likely scenarios related to the event as we can. It helps us all have a better time when Blake has a good idea of what the occasion is (bar mitzvah, birthday, school event, etc.), who we might see there (whose bar mitzvah or birthday it is, what friends and relatives will likely be there, whether there will be kids and adults), what type of food or music it will involve, whether it's likely to be noisy, and how long he should expect to be there. We also try to provide a safe, less noisy option for Blake during busy social occasions. I keep an eye on him, and if I see that he's getting agitated I might give him the choice to take a walk with me or sit in the car and watch a short DVD. These two things—a detailed preparation talk about where we're going before the event and having a safe break option while we're there—give Blake the extra support he needs to better navigate unfamiliar social situations and cut down on his frustration and confusion.

—ROSIE

child's sound and language experience grows, context changes and expands and comprehension deepens, paving the way for understanding words and assigning more nuanced and complex meanings to sounds.

AUDITORY PROCESSING DISORDERS

Most auditory processing disorders affect some combination of these four steps to good listening. Parents who can work through each of these steps as they interact with, read to, or converse with their child can help their son or daughter over some of the language and vocabulary obstacles that would otherwise make school and social life difficult in the years to come.

> Three-year-old Gary's father is reading his son a story in which one of the characters hears a joke so funny that he describes it as "hilarious." Gary's dad reads to his son often, is aware that Gary has difficulty processing language sometimes, and can tell by Gary's perplexed look that he's not familiar with the word "hilarious." The word has been detected. Gary, like many kids with APD, tends to hang on to the words he's sure of rather than seek out newer terms to broaden or focus the meanings of the things he sees, hears, and does. Humor grows and changes substantially for most children as they mature, but up to now, for Gary the word "funny" covers it all, regardless of the context. Gary's brain has made a discrimination—it hears "hilarious" but it has no comprehension of this word. If Gary does not have discrimination difficulties, he will even be able to repeat the word. He can identify what he has heard but doesn't know what it means. "I thought that was hilarious, too," Gary's dad says. "It was so funny that when the boy in the story told the joke everyone couldn't stop laughing." With help from his father, Gary can now identify what the word "hilarious" means. Later in the

story and on into dinner and at breakfast the next day, Gary's dad remembers to use the word "hilarious" a few times in conversation. When Gary describes something at supper as funny, his father asks him, "Is it funny, or is it hilarious?" and waits for an answer. In the car on the way to school the next day, Gary's dad references the word again. By hearing the word "hilarious" in multiple contexts, Gary begins to comprehend its meaning and adds it to his vocabulary, deepening his listening skills and building his stockpile of useful words.

Gary's dad successfully addressed the four steps necessary in order for listening to work:

1. *Detection.* Gary heard the word and gave a look that Gary's dad recognized indicated that his son was confused by the word "hilarious" and didn't understand what it meant.
2. *Discrimination.* Gary was able to tell the difference between the word and the sounds and words before and after it.
3. *Identification.* Gary was able to identify the unfamiliar word by its sound. He let his father know what word it was by saying it back to him. Gary's dad gave a concise description of what the word "hilarious" means in terms that Gary already knew.
4. *Comprehension.* By using the word repeatedly in conversation that night and the next day, Gary's dad gave his son a variety of contexts in which Gary's understanding of "hilarious" could deepen. Hearing the word in a new context helps Gary understand what it means.

Adding words increases the depth of vocabulary, but listening to those words being used in a variety of different experiences deepens the use and meaning of those words. In order to be helpful in preparing a child for listening and learning in school and assisting the child once he or she has reached school age, parents need to provide experiences that will enrich and deepen the child's understanding. There is so much more to the art of parenting than just making rules and setting boundaries. Equipping kids with rules, values, and a sense of the limits of acceptable responsible behavior is of course vital, but so is teaching them how to think and understand. And thinking and understanding are learned through experience.

LOOKING AT LISTENING

Even in the earliest stages of life, listening is always an active applied skill. The fine-tuned application of listening can be broken down into six distinctive qualities. The symptoms of an auditory processing disorder can manifest through any or all of these listening applications. At home and at school, there are a number of very specific things that parents and teachers can do to nurture listening and to manipulate listening environments to help a child hone listening skills. First, however, it's important to understand the six distinctive qualities.

Auditory Attention

Five-year-old Max is obsessed with trains. There are trains on the curtains in his bedroom, trains on his bedspread, and a toy box nearly overflowing with toy trains of every kind at the foot of his bed. This morning, like most mornings, Max sits at the breakfast table playing with a locomotive engine, zooming it back and forth and approximating the noise of the train whistle and engine. "Maxie," his mother asks from the next room, "would you like French toast?" Max is lost in his train game, and to him it's as if she didn't say anything. Max's mother comes to the doorway. "Max," she says less playfully, "I'm making

French toast. Would you like some?" Still Max doesn't look Finally Max's mother sharply raps the spatula she holds o tabletop and bends down low to her son's level. "Mama has a big day ahead of her at work and still needs to get everyone off to school, Max," she says impatiently. "Do you want French toast or not?" The last sentence is the first thing that Max has actually heard his mother say; in fact, it's the first thing he's heard her say since he got up out of bed. Startled by the spatula and confused by how annoyed his mother appears, he wonders why his mother is mad at him.

Auditory attention problems can be as mild as a momentary distraction. But they can also be so severe that a child has tremendous difficulty becoming aware of a sound and attending to it or focusing on it. Auditory attention is itself a skill that grows in accuracy over time and with experience. A three-year-old child can't sit focused for thirty minutes on a single sound or voice. By second grade most children can attend to and focus on a single sound, but it takes practice. Children with APDs often show a consistent inability to keep their attention on a single specific sound or voice.

Auditory Discrimination

A preschooler named Ruthie sits in her mother's lap. The two of them are making up a story about an imaginary little girl. The hero of their story has just outfoxed a mean giant and is about to claim a throne in a mountain palace. "The girl fat down," Ruthie hears her mother say, "and looked out at the room full of people she had saved." Confused, Ruthie wonders what this means. Was the little girl in the story a giant, too? Are the words "sat" and "fat" the same thing? Should she stop her mother and ask her what she meant? Distracted, Ruthie second-guesses her-

self, and her enthusiasm for making up the story wanes. Ruthie's
mother has continued the story, but Ruthie has lost interest and
tells her disappointed mom that she's too tired to continue.

Ruthie's confusion between similar-sounding words is a problem in auditory discrimination—the ability to tell the difference
between sounds. In Ruthie's case her inability to distinguish between an "f" sound and an "s" sound was enough to derail creative
story time. These distinctions become increasingly important as a
child's vocabulary and language skills grow in complexity. Children initially learn words as labels for objects. If, for instance,
"bat" and "bad" sound exactly the same, there's little chance a
child will assign the specific label "bat" to what's used in baseball.
Children who can't name things can't ask for them or offer them.
Without a useful verbal handle to put on an object or person, they
opt out of asking and offering and instead tend to grab and discard
things heedlessly. Without a clear sense of individual people's
names, jobs, or the words they can use to define or describe them,
boys and girls with auditory discrimination issues tend to withdraw from potentially fun, challenging, or educational social encounters altogether.

Learning words involves some trial and error. Perfectly intelligent adults will occasionally mispronounce words such as "library,"
"realtor," "espresso," and "nuclear" and use others incorrectly in
conversation. Children use the developmental strategy of trying
out different letter sounds and words to straighten out what something they heard is supposed to mean. A child with APD, however,
becomes locked in a constant struggle between what she hears and
what the person speaking actually intends to get across. Multiply
Ruthie's single story-halting listening error by a dozen or more a
day and you can see that problems with auditory discrimination
can be extremely rough on a child's growth and confidence. Ruthie
knows that she's wrong but doesn't know why. A child who is not

able to discriminate between word sounds and syllables finds even ordinary daily communication challenging and frustrating.

Auditory Memory

On a trip to the park with his dad, four-year-old Jason plays alongside another little boy in a sandbox. A plastic bucket and shovel set were left behind in the sandbox, and Jason and the other boy are making the most of each, while their two dads watch from a distance and talk. Tiring of using the shovel, Jason decides he'd like the bucket more. But even though his dad told him what the toy was called, he cannot remember the word his dad used. When the two children started playing together his dad also told Jason what the other little boy's name was. But Jason can't really remember what that was, either. Jason tries pointing at the bucket and pointing at the other little boy, but that doesn't help. Finally Jason simply tries to grab the bucket away—making his would-be new friend cry, and earning a scolding from his dad.

Without the basic skill of auditory memory, communicating specifically and clearly is nearly impossible. Even under the best circumstances, information we acquire from listening fades quickly from our short-term or working memory. If a child like Jason can't hold sound information in his brain's "in-box" long enough to assign meaning to it, he'll have a difficult time using language. Our brains make a more permanent place for the words and sounds we hear repeatedly. Jason, who has difficulty processing sound through memory, can barely recall each individual instance of hearing a word, and his vocabulary suffers as a result. Without the words on hand to describe how he feels or what he wants, Jason has to take matters into his own hands or do without.

Auditory Sequential Memory

> While out in their backyard garden together, five-year-old
> Tracey asks her mother if she can help her as she tends to a rose-
> bush. "Sure, honey," her mother replies, "that would be very
> nice. Can you put this stone in the wheelbarrow, and get me the
> watering can and the hose?" Tracey's mother hands her daugh-
> ter a small smooth stone and Tracey rushes off to where the
> wheelbarrow, watering can, and garden hose lie alongside each
> other a few yards away. When Tracey comes back she is still
> holding the stone, has dragged the garden hose with her and left
> the watering can where it was. "I need the watering can, too,"
> her mother says. "And didn't I ask you to put the stone in the
> wheelbarrow?"

A request of the complexity of the one that Tracey's mother
made should not be out of the reach of a five-year-old. But if a
child's brain has difficulty processing auditory information sequentially, a carefully laid-out sequence of instructions can become a jumble. The individual words in a sentence become
confused, switched around, and impossible to use as a road map
indicating what to do or say next. Sequential memory is really a
parallel skill to auditory memory. Memory captures individual
bits of information, and sequential memory allows us to remember them in a meaningful order. Numbers, letters, and the pronounced tones and sounds and rhythm of speech cease to have
meaning if we can't recall them in a connected chain of order that
allows them to make sense.

Children chunk together increasingly complex bits of heard
information as they grow. The glue that holds that information
together—a sentence, a rhyme, a series of instructions, a
melody—is the recalled sequence the information arrives in. A
child who cannot keep auditory information in order is lost in

conversations and social interactions, cannot follow instructions, and is denied a vital skill for making math and reading possible.

Auditory Figure/Ground

Jonah sits quietly in his first-grade classroom. At the front of the classroom his teacher describes the permission slip that parents will need to fill out for a field trip scheduled for the following week. Outside the classroom window, a custodian starts up a lawn mower. In the next seat one of Jonah's classmates whispers to the young student seated behind Jonah. A chair squeaks loudly as another student shifts in his seat. Jonah looks up and realizes that the teacher is now standing in front of his desk. "Is that all clear to everyone?" she asks, and then adds, smiling down, "Jonah, do you have any questions?" Jonah realizes he has no idea what the topic is, let alone what questions to ask. Rather than embarrass himself, he simply shakes his head and hopes he can figure out later what the teacher was talking about.

The act of listening requires us to prioritize sounds constantly. We can't hold everything there is to hear around us in focus at all times. Something has to be the front-and-center sound we listen to. This constant prioritizing and arrangement of the sounds around us is called auditory figure/ground. A child who struggles with figure/ground is unable to separate sounds, decide which is the most important one, and then direct and concentrate his or her attention on that sound. Most of the students in Jonah's class naturally register each sound—the teacher's voice, the lawn mower, the classmate's whisper, and the chair squeak—as either a foreground sound or a background sound. A child with an APD is often unable to sort out two or more sounds and establish and maintain that foreground/background relationship. This child will gravitate toward the source of each new sound, no matter where it comes from, confusing the essential with the nonessential and letting low-priority sounds come forward into the auditory foreground to obscure the sound that he should attend to. Unaccustomed to the teacher-first hierarchy of sound in a classroom, such a child risks becoming academically stranded. Over time, as a child without figure/ground skills acts on what little he has gleaned from the rules and behavioral expectations laid out by his teachers, he can seem demanding and disruptive.

Auditory Cohesion

Libby, a first grader, is trying to fit in as best she can with an energetic group of other little girls at school. "Knock knock," one of Libby's classmates says for the fifth time to the group. All of the girls except Libby chime in once again with, "Who's there?"

"Banana!" says the first girl, a little more exaggeratedly than the previous four times. Libby looks around wide-eyed. She feeds on the social energy and enthusiasm everyone shares but is worried because she doesn't really know what everyone is so giddy about.

"Banana who?" the other girls exclaim, anticipating a payoff that has Libby completely baffled.

"Knock knock," the first girl says with an emphasis, making it clear to everyone but Libby that this is the last time.

"Who's there?" everyone but Libby shouts in unison. Libby fights an urge to join in by telling them all that it's probably banana!

"Orange!" the first girl laughs.

"Orange who?" the others roar.

"Orange you glad I didn't say banana!" Everyone but Libby howls with girlish laughter. When the laughter subsides Libby looks at one of her classmates and quietly asks, "What happened to banana?" The other little girls ignore Libby and race off together following the first girl to the swings. Libby remains behind, feeling foolish and trying to figure out what just happened. Maybe her mom and dad can explain it later, she thinks as she watches her classmates play together.

Once a growing child masters perceiving, identifying, recalling, placing in sequence, and prioritizing a string of sounds as language, the brain opens up words into the many different ways that they can be used, pronounced, and intended. Auditory cohesion makes it possible to choose one of the many different strands of meaning that trail sounds, words, and the way they are said. Verbal communication is like doing a three-dimensional jigsaw puzzle. Handed a jumble of possibilities, our brains examine that information, gauging the specific words spoken, how they fit together, the pitch, rhythm, and tone with which they were offered, the expression of the person saying them, and dozens of other defining details. The way those individual qualities line up and fit together conveys meaning.

Auditory cohesion puts all those pieces together. Double meanings, irony, words such as "pair" and "pear" that sound the same but mean distinctly different things, understatement, verbal humor, idioms, subtext, and inference—all these are possible only when the brain's auditory cortex is able to bring cohesion into the mix to make it all work. A child who doesn't develop auditory cohesion skills on schedule is confused by figurative language and intentional absurdities. Her inability to reach beyond the first level of language skills also denies her humor and wordplay and the means to make sense of indirect or veiled requests. Delivered with the right inference, the sentence "It's a little hot in here, don't you think?" can be a deliberate attempt at getting someone to open a window. A kid with APD may have trouble just under-

standing the words "little" and "hot" used together, let alone realizing that she's being asked to perform a task. When you consider
how much of learning and social interaction relies on abstract
language, it becomes important to recognize that the cohesion
skills necessary to lift language from the merely literal are vital.

PART TWO

COPING DAILY WITH APD

FOUR

A Sound Strategy for Moving Ahead

P arents hold the keys to a world in which a child confidently uses his natural abilities to their fullest. But to use those keys effectively, parents need facts and strategies. Raising and nurturing a child in a way that allows the child to take full advantage of his natural capabilities is a complex process that unfolds in an ever-changing environment, and tracing the entirety of this process is beyond the scope of any one book. Yet helpful and useful information is all around us. It just doesn't come from a single source. Books such as this one, expert advice from educators and from other parents in person and on the Internet, and information you get from observing how your child reacts to different situations all present opportunities to gain useful knowledge of how listening develops, how listening impacts language, and how listening and language development in turn impact learning. Equipped with a body of knowledge and an ongoing desire to add to it, you can offer your child a well-balanced "auditory diet" of enlivening sounds, music, and human speech. If your child has an auditory processing disorder—or you suspect that he does—expanding your body of knowledge about how listening skills are formed and differentiated will serve you well.

Giving any child the best advantages toward achieving his listening and social potential takes planning. Cultivating and integrating smart sound strategies and implementing even subtle changes in an auditory situation can make a tremendous difference in any child's ability to attend to the right sounds and listen well. Sound strategies are the difference between raising a child in an environment that fosters openness and success versus one that reinforces the anger and frustration of being trapped in an overwhelming sound environment.

Most children with APD aren't really aware that they have trouble processing information. They feel that they can hear as well as everyone else and that they understand the messages and words they encounter. What they do know is that they're not getting the right reactions—approval, feelings of accomplishment, emotional bonds with the people with whom they communicate. That only leaves themselves to blame. Constant frustration has a devastating effect on a child's self-esteem. "Other kids get it," "I still don't understand," "But that's what you wanted me to do," and other words of disappointment and rejection replace the exuberant expressions of enthusiasm and positive feelings that other kids share. The first and most important strategy to adopt with a child who has an APD—at any age—is to lovingly support the child as you work together. Let your child know:

- *She is not "dumb."* Going on playdates, going to school, and participating in extracurricular activities come with a lot of painful experiences for children struggling with an APD. Over time, your child can begin to feel incompetent and start to believe that her siblings, friends, or classmates who don't struggle with listening skills are smarter than she is.

APD and many other auditory obstacles have nothing to do with intelligence. Don't give your child permission to feel less intelligent than her peers and refer to herself as "dumb" or "stupid." Remind your child that everyone learns in different ways and struggles to make sense of things sometimes. Make sure to talk through situations or moments that are baffling or confusing to both of you, so that your child understands that "not getting it" happens to everyone.

- *She is not alone.* Children with APD often think they are the only ones wrestling with sound. Point out when you cannot hear well in noisy environments and describe how it makes you feel. Explain to your child that everyone has trouble listening in certain places and gets frustrated, and that it's perfectly fine to ask for help.
- *She is noticed . . . and loved.* Don't pass up opportunities to praise your child's natural strengths and reward her accomplishments. Children need pride, purpose, and a feeling that they are loved. Reasonable and honest praise will make all the difference to them.

SOUND CHOICES

It can sometimes seem as if we are at cross purposes with our kids. But children and parents really want the same things. No child wants to be unsuccessful at school and unhappy at home. I've worked with hundreds of children with auditory difficulties and I've never met a single one who had a genuine desire to fail. Life is all about choice, and it's parents' responsibility to teach their children how to make positive choices in their lives. A child with an APD can feel as if he has no choices and no control. While he may not be able to control his APD, he still has the power of choice.

Both of you share the power to create environments that are conducive to listening and to listen better in situations that are less than ideal for communicating and learning. Successfully dealing with APD difficulties at home, at school, and out in the larger world requires a team effort. It takes a combination of your efforts to adapt a sound environment and advocate on behalf of your child and your child's own ability to adapt and apply what he understands about difficult listening environments to achieve lasting success.

Having an undiagnosed or untreated APD builds walls around children. Kids who have had continuing trouble listening may also have continuing trouble adapting and trying out new things. They tend to keep those walls up and naturally resist change. Your child needs to understand why you are asking him to make certain changes. He also has to feel that he is being set up for success, an experience that for a child with APD can seem much less familiar than failure. Help your child to understand that success is cause and effect, not a roll of the dice or something that just "happens" to some kids, and that the choices your child makes and the strategies he uses to compensate for his auditory challenges are a major part of what causes success. Your child needs to believe he is part of a team that is focused on finding solutions. Together, the two of you will lead a group effort by partnering with the people in your lives who can also facilitate your child's progress.

Take the time to speak with siblings, extended family members, friends, other parents, babysitters, day care workers, school bus drivers, teachers, counselors, coaches, and others who regularly interact with your child. Share the strategies and facts that you've learned about your child's APD and how to deal with it. Some parents come to believe that explaining a child's individual needs to others, especially relative strangers, is burdensome or an unnecessary airing of private concerns. Actually, the opposite is true. Leaving the people who care about your child or are charged with looking after him to discover what your child is and isn't capable of on their own puts much more of a burden on them and ultimately will add to your child's frustration. Most people will be willing to adapt to your child's needs once they understand the unique challenges of his listening disorder.

By reaching out, explaining what your child's needs are, and getting the cooperation of the people in your child's life, you are in effect creating a nurturing and supportive shawl or blanket that will extend into every part of the growing community of people with whom your child interacts on a daily basis.

LISTENING AT HOME

The job of helping relieve your child of some of the burden of APD begins with the home environment itself. Teachers and therapists can work wonders with children who have listening difficulties, but every day begins and ends at home. Dealing with APD needs to be part of home life, too. Home is under your jurisdiction and control. You need to be aware of what you can do to make it a safe haven for a child who is frustrated and challenged by listening to and understanding language in the world outside of her house. A good way to keep that in mind is to answer the following questions.

What's Going On Around the Two of You?

Giving directions, explaining something, reading a story—no matter what it is, if you're trying to verbally engage your child, you need to take stock of where you are doing it. Is there a television on? Is there a radio or CD playing? Are there other conversations going on nearby? Is the room small enough that your child and you are facing each other? Do you have your daughter's attention? Is she looking at you as well as listening to what you're saying? Sharing a quiet room uncluttered by TV and other sounds helps a child's comprehension enormously.

Are You Really Listening to Each Other?

Not being understood and heard is incredibly isolating and difficult for a child. If you can make it clear that you hear and understand her, it will reduce the frustration your child feels with much
of the rest of the world. Simplify your language and speak as
plainly as you can until you recognize that your child is getting
what you're saying. Follow closely what she says in return, and
don't be afraid to ask simple questions to clarify what she is trying to tell you.

Are You Meeting on a Level Playing Field?

When giving directions or supervising activities with your child,
scale back your expectations. Don't make every situation a test of
whether or not he can follow orders or do what you tell him to do.
Give one direction at a time and ask your child to repeat back
what you said so that you can gauge how much he understood.
For some children with APD the simple and familiar instructions
"Go put on your pajamas. Time to brush your teeth. Let's get a
book to read" may be too ambitious a series of tasks to absorb at
once, even if they can successfully do each step separately. It helps
tremendously to break strings of activities down into individual
steps and get confirmation from the child as each one is done.
"Let's go upstairs . . . here we are. Got your pajamas? Put 'em on.
Okay? Let's go to the sink. Where's that toothbrush?" Take your
time, and leave pauses between words and directions so that your
child can successfully sort out each task individually.

Are You Keeping Your Language Down to Earth?

Your child's ability to process more sophisticated language will
grow as you nurture her listening and comprehension skills, but

I'm an artist and I tend to speak in metaphors. But Blake is a kid whose thinking is very literal. Metaphors can be hard for him to comprehend meaningfully. If I say to him, "You are really getting to be too big for your britches," he's likely to respond, "What are you talking about? I am not on a bridge." If a teacher says something like "Don't paint yourself into a corner," he'll point out that he doesn't even have a paintbrush. For Blake, much of life and conversation is factual and literal. I have to strip away flowery descriptions and ironies when we talk, pare things down to the basic bare facts, and go from there.

—ROSIE

no matter the age at which you discover an auditory processing disorder, it is good to bring your language down a notch or two while you are trying to get a handle on what specifically trips up your child. Avoid similes ("You run like the wind"), metaphors ("It's raining cats and dogs"), sarcasm ("No, your *other* left"), and intentionally misleading word choices if your child has difficulty understanding complex language. Save abstract ideas, verbal humor, and double meanings for teaching-time sessions. Hearing simple, straight, unambiguous words is a huge relief for a child with APD. The clearer you are, the easier it is for the child to understand what you're doing together, meet your expectations, and not become frustrated.

Are You Making Sure That You Were Understood?

A child with APD does not always know when he didn't hear something correctly. Asked, "Do you understand?" or "Did you hear me?" such a child will often say yes because he believes he did. He heard something—it just may not have been complete or coherent to him. A better way to confirm that you were understood is to ask the child about what happens next based on what you've said to him. Instead of asking if he heard you say, "Wash your hands for supper" or "Time for your bath," ask the child what he is going to do now. The answer to that question will give a clear idea of whether you were heard and understood. If his answer is correct, the child can then follow through. If it's incorrect, you have the opportunity to repeat and rephrase the instruction or statement and give your child a chance to be successful.

Are You Clear on Why Your Child Acted Out?

Try to learn to recognize the difference between difficulty listening and stubbornness, acting out, or tantrums. Is a moment of trouble or a tendency toward difficult behavior due to APD? Rushing to judgment before checking in with your child to see if she heard you correctly will only frustrate both of you. So many times I have seen a child proudly finish a chore thinking she was following the direction perfectly, only to be told, "You weren't listening!"

Are You Passing On What You're Learning About Listening Environments?

As you work together, you'll begin to get a sense of what sound environments are suitable for your child to practice the skill of listening. Pass it along. Teach your child how to become aware of listening situations that may be difficult for him, and share strategies for choosing environments that will allow him to hear and understand sounds better. "Maybe you're having trouble understanding because you can't hear who's talking, honey," a mother might point out. "What do you think might happen if you changed seats so you could hear better?" Moving, asking permission to change seats, or asking to turn off a TV set, fan, or other source of background noise will remind your child that he always has choices.

WAYS TO WORK

A child's listening and language skills naturally grow based on her exposure to quality sound stimulation. Every time you speak and listen to your child, you are conducting a lesson. Intentionally or not, whether at home or in the car, at dinner or at bedtime, while reading a story to your child or asking how her day was, you are demonstrating how to fine-tune her listening skills. Every parent needs to be aware of this responsibility. A child's developmental appetite for language and sound needs feeding. Throughout the day, no matter how mundane or off-the-cuff the activity, when you speak and listen together you are feeding that appetite.

Make Listening and Learning Fun and an Everyday Activity

No matter how much your child may enjoy school, it's still a child's job—his work. After working hard all day in school, your child will probably want to come home and relax. Depending on what the speech pathologist has told you, the kinds of listening lessons you and your child do together are probably best incorporated into daily living activities such as cooking, chores, bedtime reading, and so on. The goal is to make building listening skills as much fun as possible. Since you're working together to make listening second nature, you should go about it as naturally and pleasantly as you can.

The Right Shared Listening Space

Set up a listening environment within your home that's as quiet as you can arrange. In modern homes, it's often hard to find a room or space that's both quiet and free of visual distractions and foot traffic. Over the years I've learned to pick a space that has as neutral a sound and look as possible. Echoey or noisy spaces, brightly colored rooms, or rooms with large windows can distract from the job of listening. I've worked with children in bedrooms, parents' home offices, rec rooms, basements, laundry rooms, hallways that aren't used much, even bathrooms when that's the most quiet room available.

- Turn off any audible TVs and radios and make sure the phone's ringer is off.
- Sit next to your child so that she will concentrate on sound rather than on your expressions.
- Try to sit with your backs to open doors, busy patterned wall coverings, mirrors, and so on, to minimize visual distractions.
- Work at a table, with the book, toys, game, or pictures you're using in front of the two of you.

WAYS TO PLAY

Chapter 9 details the inherent benefits of unstructured play for children with APD (indeed, for all children). Working with games and activities that pair sounds and language with visual aids such as toys, pictures, or written words and sentences is a recipe for success for kids with APD. As your child grows more successful, phase out visually cued activities in favor of auditory-only activities.

- Try not to unnecessarily repeat directions or a word you want the child to listen to. Instead, pause after individual instructions or words and give your child a chance to process what you've said and then respond.
- Praise is important—reinforce success. "Great, let's try it again," "Wow," and "Yes" all send a succinct positive message.
- Overpraising is counterproductive. Telling your child he is "the smartest little boy in the whole wide world!" shifts focus from your child's feeling successful at a given task to his working toward praise and approval alone. You'll recognize how much praise is enough for your child.
- Follow a time limit. Don't overwork each other. Listening is difficult and inherently exhausting for a child with APD. Begin with ten to fifteen minutes per activity and try to end before it's clear that your child needs it to end.
- Start with success. At first your child will probably need to make a connection between word and image in order to understand things. It's important to begin on a successful note to build enthusiasm, so use pictures as much as is necessary initially. If you start with no visual reference, your child's listening weakness may make the chosen activity more of a test than a game. Always begin where the child can meet success and then slowly increase the level of difficulty. The learning process may seem slow, but when a child is successful, information is stored better.

FIVE

The Art of Noise:
Creating Better Listening Environments

Close your eyes and the world of sight and vision vanishes. Now "close your ears"—consciously try to turn off the sensation of sound and the hearing and listening your ears and brain do together. It's not so easy, is it? If you're not eating or hungry, you don't really experience a constant baseline sensation of taste. Unless you are wearing an itchy or irritating fabric or you've been soaked in the rain, you don't have a recurring touch sensation of your clothes on your skin. Four of the five senses can be compared to air-conditioning—you don't notice them unless something is wrong. But hearing never stops.

The shifting overlap of conversations, music, and the natural noises and tones we encounter throughout the day is a garden of multiple delights and varied experiences. Sometimes those sounds can become exhausting and stressful. Much as we may wish it were otherwise, the sense of hearing lacks an off switch. We can close our eyes and to varying degrees turn off our other senses, but our ears are always open for business.

Dealing with the constant unnecessary stimulation of a loud and complex sound environment is frequently overtaxing, annoying, or distracting to adults. For a child, it can be overwhelming. Children do not always have the words available to communicate their confusion or discomfort. They also lack the experience necessary to actively seek clarity and quiet, eliminate conflicting sound sources, or move to a less chaotic auditory situation. A chaotic sound environment pushes children into the borderland between acceptable and unacceptable behavior. Stressed by circumstances beyond their control, children will react by acting out—crying, becoming irritable, acting silly, withdrawing, or offering little or no attention. Some children are simply more sensitive to sound than others. The combination of that sensitivity and an inability to do anything to protect themselves and compensate for a listening-hostile environment can make children frustrated and angry to the point that they appear to have behavioral issues.

Children with an APD or other auditory difficulties are particularly vulnerable to the extremes of sounds around them. As you'll remember from Chapter 3, a child with APD may struggle with figure/ground—the listening ability that allows us to sort, prioritize, and arrange sounds so that we are able to listen. For children with figure/ground problems and other APD symptoms, noise can be the auditory equivalent of a blindfold. Just as a person with a blindfold is forced to take awkward, tentative steps and feel around in front of him, a child with APD stumbles and struggles in a noisy auditory arena while trying to make his way in conversations and other necessary listening.

Any situation or experience can present a sound environment full of obstacles for a child with an APD. Since there's no set specific cure for APD, you and your child will need to learn to stay a step ahead, see potential problems coming, and assess the possibility for difficulty and confusion in the environments you encounter. Once the two of you understand where your child experiences the greatest difficulty processing auditory information, you can work together on creating and sharing better listening environments.

NOTICING THE NOISE AROUND YOU

If we could see sound waves in the air the way we see ripples, waves, and bubbles in water, everything before us would be revealed as part of a complex and ever-changing sound environment. Each surface, object, and person we encounter is generating sound, reflecting and bouncing sound around, absorbing, transforming, or transferring its vibrations in varying combinations and intensities. This constant bombardment of primary sounds, reflections, ripples, and competing sound sources can be one of the great pleasures of the sensory world.

The subtle background sound of outside air circulating through a window, people talking at various distances and volumes, telephones ringing, music blaring or playing quietly in the distance, sudden noises such as dogs barking, doors slamming, or car alarms going off—our brains are always sifting, sorting, and comparing the countless voices, noises, and sounds that we encounter every day. People with typical auditory capabilities have an internal mechanism that organizes and prioritizes sounds, putting background noise and monotonous, irrelevant noises on the back burner and helping us to keep up front what we're really listening to. But when we encounter a sound environment where background noise and foreground sound are similar in volume and tone, that prioritizing becomes difficult and sometimes even impossible. In a situation where sounds cancel one another out, we're forced to compensate as best we can. We'll lean forward to single out a speaker and use our eyes to catch visual cues such as facial expressions, gestures, or lip movements that may help us make sense of what we're hearing. We'll make choices and take action to lessen the conflicting noise, or we'll abandon the situation and try to find a quieter place in which we can successfully listen.

On your way to becoming an adult who can listen, use language, and communicate effectively, you have traveled the same developmental path as your child. You have experienced the frustration of not being heard, of losing track of a voice or a sound you want or need to hear in an enveloping soundscape of extraneous noise. Though you can handle a lot of sound at once, your attention has its limits, too. Noise fights listening whenever there are too many individual overlapping signals competing for our auditory attention. A noisy environment is like an old-fashioned switchboard in which all the circuits are in use and no more information can get through. Most of us can patiently sort out and filter background noises so that we can concentrate on the signal we want to hear. Children, especially children with APD, learn these skills of listening over time. Some struggle with it constantly and need to be taught and reminded what they should be listening to and what they need to ignore.

Really noisy environments mask the familiar and reassuring sound of your speaking voice so well that your child can feel ignored or abandoned and left to cope in an arena she's years away from mastering. Unless you understand when this is happening to your child, you will find navigating loud and noisy sound environments a constant tug-of-war between your desire to communicate with your child and her limited ability to meaningfully perceive what you are trying to do.

Take a moment to think about situations in which sound is challenging for you, then think about ones that may be challenging for your child. Watch, observe, and ask your child how she's doing and feeling when the two of you are together in new or difficult sound environments. Make note of the places where she seems to have the most trouble listening or is the most uncomfortable trying to attend to you and to what's going on around you. Your home, family car, the school bus and public transportation, airports, train stations, restaurants, movie theaters, the supermarket, stores, and malls can all be sources of suffocating and frustrating noise for some children. Bear in mind that just because an environment is supposed to be "kid-friendly" doesn't guarantee that it's listening-friendly. Playgrounds, amusement parks, kid-themed restaurants and activity centers, circuses, aquariums and zoos, a relative's or friend's house, and even the children's room at the library may appear inviting, but crowded spaces, multiple voices, constant sound, TVs, loudspeakers, and bright lights can be bewildering to your child.

All this is not to say that you should withdraw from going out in public with your child or swear off anything involving lots of sound or potential for noise. Rather, you should simply consider the destinations your family chooses in terms of how they sound and what effect that sound may have on your child. Think about your expectations for your child. Instead of trying to figure out what went wrong after a bad sound environment experience, ask yourself these questions beforehand.

- What are you expecting of your child?
- Are you facing a potentially noisy situation?
- Is what you are expecting too difficult for your child?
- What can you potentially change about this situation?
- How can you adapt this listening environment to make it a more fun and pleasurable experience for your child?

Preparation and patience are key. Before going on an outing where noise may present a problem for you and your child, talk the trip over with your child first. Let her know in advance where you are going. Preview the trip—traveling, getting there, what to expect when you arrive, when you're likely to leave, and when you'll be coming home. Use vocabulary that is familiar and positive, and patiently answer any questions your child has no matter how trivial they may seem. Your child wants to have fun and spend time with you. When you come to an understanding about what the possibilities are on a family outing, you let your child know that what lies ahead is an opportunity for fun, not something risky or scary.

Plans change, things come up, and details and destinations can get altered at the last minute. If you've been prepared for a trip and circumstances force you to change your schedule or cancel, just make that part of the experience. Life is constant change, and though young children and children with an APD in particular resist change, exposing them to some of life's randomness and compromise will prepare them to cope with more of it later in life. Reasonable change is good. It helps children to become more flexible, rather than imprisoned by the way they think things "should" be.

Even a modest amount of preparation and attending to sound issues in your child's life will pay tremendous rewards by reducing short-term frustrations and increasing long-term benefits.

HOME AND FAMILY

Dealing effectively with noise begins in the home. Perform an inventory of the rooms in your house or apartment. What makes it noisy? Do your floors and doors squeak? Do chairs scrape? Does an individual room have a high ceiling or hard surfaces that harshly reflect sound, or is it close to the sound of street traffic? Note the times of day when noisy activity is at its peak. Once you've established where and when things can be kept quiet, use that place and time to pass on particularly important information or spend quality time with your child. Remember that yelling directions from one room to another is never a good strategy. If you need to talk to your child, go to where he is and face him. When you and your child need to communicate, turn off or get away from loud appliances such as the dishwasher or the TV. Family meals can be hectic under any circumstances. Explore strategies to keep dinnertime noise as low as is practical, such as reminding your children to speak politely and not interrupt, or putting food on plates in the kitchen rather than passing and serving at the table. What are the best ways to communicate when the family is together? A little observation will tell you a lot. Discuss what APD is with all your children and anyone else under your roof. After you've all made any accommodations you need to for a child with APD, be sure to treat everyone in the family equally. Maintain the same expectations about behavior and interest in the activities of all the children in your family.

Cars

Families that spend a lot of time driving from one activity to the next need to choose with extra care where a child with an APD sits. Children with auditory differences usually listen better on one side or the other. If this is true of your child, make sure she sits in a seat that positions the stronger ear toward your voice and the weaker ear closer to a window. Trial and error is the best way to figure out how best to use the car. Putting two or three children together in the backseat and leaving the front passenger seat empty, for instance, may make for a more difficult listening environment than is necessary. Air-conditioning, open windows, music, and showing DVDs all contribute competing noise. They may make conversations difficult to hold and directions difficult to follow for a child with APD.

Restaurants

Nine-year-old Henry is barely hanging on. When his mom and dad announced that afternoon that they were taking the family out to dinner, Henry hoped that they meant they were going to his favorite place, a Mexican restaurant. Something about the big booths, soft seats, thick carpets, and mild-mannered people who worked there always made him feel safer and happy when his family ate there on special occasions. But the new pub that his family chose is making Henry miserable. From the minute his family arrived Henry felt assaulted by the incessant clinking of cups and plates, whirring blenders, hissing espresso machine, customers laughing and talking loudly, pounding music, and staff shouting orders to and from the noisy open kitchen.

Henry's family is enjoying the excitement that charges the air. They talk and tell jokes as they wait for their hamburgers. But, seated with his back to a wall at a corner table, Henry can't make out what everyone is talking about and what is making them laugh. Finally, bored and frustrated, he lets his head drop to the table. Henry's mother takes his arm and tells him to sit up and act his age. He doesn't want to ruin the evening for everyone, but he doesn't want to be ignored or punished for feeling bad, either. Henry's behavior gets worse as the evening wears on, until finally his parents decide to leave the restaurant early. It is supposed to be punishment, but for a nine-year-old boy with APD, it feels like relief.

It's a fact of physics that sound bounces off hard surfaces and dissipates in high-ceilinged rooms and that nearby voices can lose clarity and effectiveness in an environment hosting multiple competing background noises. A crowded restaurant can pose a nearly

insurmountable auditory challenge to a child with an APD. High
ceilings, brick and glass walls, and hardwood floors combine with
the sound of cutlery, piped-in or live music, bustling staff, kitchen
noise, and dozens of people speaking simultaneously from different parts of the room to create a perfect storm of auditory confusion for a child sensitive to sound. It can be a challenge for adults
to communicate effectively in restaurants with terrible acoustics,
but children with auditory difficulties can find the experience
frustrating, annoying, and even terrifying.

A few commonsense rules can help you and your child get the
most out of treats such as family restaurant trips on special occasions and while on vacation.

- Take note of which restaurants and other places appear to
  frustrate your child. Either choose other restaurants or prepare your child for the experience in advance and make
  sure to pay attention to her needs while you are there.
- Choose quieter, less crowded parts of restaurants when possible. Note the proximity to loudspeakers, kitchen en-
  trances, and noisy equipment such as cash registers or
  coffeemakers, and ask for a table that's not located near
  anything loud.
- Ask to be seated in soft banquettes or against walls with
  cloth wall coverings when possible.
- Find out what your child wants to order before you leave
  the house so that she can be ready to communicate with the
  server. Review the menu in advance. Most restaurants are
  happy to e-mail or fax a copy of their menu, and many have
  their menus available online.
- Let your child participate in choosing the restaurant. She
  may want to try a new place even if the environment pre-
  sents greater listening challenges. The fact that she had a
  say will incline her to try harder to enjoy herself.

There's a theme-y kind of restaurant here in town where they have sports and TV and video games, and it's kind of noisy. Before we understood what Blake was going through, we would go there and Blake would sulk and sort of put his head down and say he didn't want to order anything. We came to realize that the noise level in that place is so intense for him that he had to shut everything off. So we don't go to that restaurant anymore. We make sure to have a quiet place to eat or a place where he is able to participate in the conversation. We're very destination-oriented at the mall now, too. We don't wander. We get exactly what we need and then we leave.

—ROSIE

MAKING CHANGES AT SCHOOL

A classroom should be a place where a child is able to learn and to have fun without having to struggle to listen. If competing noises interfere with your child's ability to focus on and attend to what his teachers are saying, he'll lose the desire to pay attention and learn. Once again, preparation is the key to success. Ask your child's teachers to provide a list of subjects, themes, and vocabulary words your child will be studying, to give you an idea of the approach the teacher intends to take in class. Use this information to familiarize yourself with what your child has in store for him during the school year. Children with APD and other auditory difficulties find it easier to listen and to pay attention when they are already familiar with key concepts and vocabulary words they'll be asked to use. Classroom achievement feels a lot more possible when a child has some idea of what to expect and what's expected of him. Equipped with the basics, he can immediately focus on the lesson at hand and move forward by linking new in-

SCHOOL MEETINGS

Aparent's informed advocacy on behalf of his or her child is simply vital. If your child has been diagnosed with APD or identified as having a listening disorder, contact your school and ask to set up a meeting with your child's teachers, counselors, and any other specialists and school personnel who will be working with or instructing your child that year. Anyone at your child's school who interacts directly with your child will be able to do a better job once he or she understands the disorder, how it affects your child, and what classroom and school accommodations can help.

Persistence will pay off. School administrators often feel that they have the answers already, and sometimes they do. The usual initial official response to a meeting request may be, "We know how to handle this issue." Your child's school may very well have taught children with auditory challenges before, but the specifics of how APD affects learning are varied and highly individual. Your school may have learned how to support a child with a completely different set of symptoms from your child's.

Parents take the point position when working with schools, but educators need input from other professionals to make choices and arrangements that will work for everyone. Once you convince your school of the necessity for a meeting, make sure that the speech-language pathologist or audiologist you have consulted or are working with attends the meeting and maps out an agenda.

The school needs to be told:

- The type of disorder or challenge your child has
- How it is expressed in your child

- What accommodations can be made
- That helping your child to achieve his or her full learning and social potential at school requires a team effort

Recommendations and possibilities need to be discussed, such as:

- Reducing noise in the classroom
- Preferential seating so that your child can see and hear the teacher
- Possibly using amplification equipment for your child, such as a personal FM receiver or a sound field system (which amplifies a teacher's voice through a wireless transmitter and allows every child in a classroom to hear equally)
- Using closed captioning on videos and DVDs shown in class

I've attended hundreds of these meetings, and each one has been a win-win situation for everyone concerned. Teachers appreciate the information they get about a child's needs, and both child and parent gain additional respect for a school that is supportive and willing to listen.

formation he discovers in class with the prior knowledge he got from the preview at home.

A speech-language pathologist can prescribe a good course to follow when trying to give an individual child with an APD the advantages he'll need to fully participate in school. While actual recommendations need to be made by your child's speech-language therapist, any of the following suggestions may help your child to listen more effectively in the classroom. These guidelines can also assist teachers in creating and sustaining an educational environment in which each child in the class has an equal opportunity to learn.

Preferential Seating

Desks that are located close to the teacher and offer a good view of the teacher's face and as many other students as possible will help a child to listen effectively. Seating a child away from distracting noise sources such as hallway doors, open windows, electric pencil sharpeners, air conditioners, and heaters is also a must.

Communication Strategies

Teachers also need their own strategies to help students with APD listen and learn better. Your child's teacher should:

- Repeat announcements that are made over the PA system
- Alert a student with an APD when he or she is about to give important information by calling the child's name, making direct eye contact, or pointing to an ear as a signal to listen
- Repeat or rephrase questions and comments from other students in the classroom, especially when children are mumbling or all speaking at once
- Implement a one-voice rule and only accept responses by recognizing raised hands in the classroom
- Point to the student who has the floor and remember to call him or her by name (particularly helpful for children who have difficulty localizing sounds—they may not be able to tell which direction another student's voice is coming from,

but they'll learn to identify names with seating and know who is speaking)

- Avoid speaking to the class or giving out important information while writing on the blackboard
- Communicate clearly and energetically without exaggerating his or her speech
- Avoid moving around the room while talking
- Be patient and pause for a few moments after asking a child with APD a question, giving the child extra time to process information
- Be willing to rephrase a sentence or simplify instructions to single steps

Communication Checks

Teachers who have had success teaching students with APD use communication checks to avoid miscommunication. Instead of asking, "Did you hear me?" or "Do you understand what I said?" a teacher will check in directly with a child when important directions are given and ask, "What are you going to do?" This gives the student a chance to repeat back what she heard the way that she heard it. If what the child says is accurate and addresses what the teacher said, they can move on. But if the child understood only part of what was said, the teacher now has an opportunity to fill in any blanks and correct any wrong information. Communication checks like this are a highly effective strategy for dealing with students who have APD and tend to miss individual words or key details.

Visual Support

Adding a visual element to class activities gives students with APD another way to take in the lesson being taught and supports what they are hearing. Teachers who write assignments and other important information on the blackboard and use pictures and other visual aids to back up what they're saying engage children with auditory challenges by appealing to two senses at once. At the same time, permitting visual distractions in a classroom—clutter, excess movement, irregular traffic in and out of the room—makes it hard for students with APD to stay focused. Keeping walls and shelves neat and foot traffic to a minimum makes for a better learning environment.

REDUCING NOISE IN ALL ENVIRONMENTS

If you think back to your early school years, you can probably recall the tidal wave of sound typical of the early grades. Bells, laughter, footsteps, slammed doors, squeaking chairs—most schools, and most homes, are set up to generate noise, not to quell it. Both your home and your child's classroom likely have hard surfaces, windows, thin walls, and other acoustic properties that are potential liabilities for a child with an APD. Fortunately, there are simple ways to make schools and homes better places to learn. These easy and inexpensive changes can drastically reduce the noise level at home and in your child's classroom.

- Close windows and doors during class or during reading and wordplay time at home.
- Use felt pads, slit tennis balls, or Hushh-ups sound deadeners for the bottoms of chair legs at home and school, or see if your child's school will purchase Hushh-ups for the classroom.
- Try to replace fluorescent bulbs, which tend to hum and buzz, with incandescent lights.
- Lubricate doors and windows that squeak.
- Wear soft-soled shoes around the house and suggest that teachers and students at your child's school do the same.

Lois suggested that we buy these Hushh-up things, which are like tennis balls that go on the bottoms of all the chairs. They eliminate the squeaky noise that happens when you move a chair. I'll be honest with you—I didn't think it would make a difference, but it has totally changed things. It's even affected my ability to be calm in the house, too. You don't realize how much extra noise that kind of thing makes until it's gone.

—ROSIE

- Soften hard sound-reflective surfaces such as tile or linoleum floors, brick walls, and banks of windows by installing carpets, drapes, self-adhesive corkboards, or acoustic tiles.

As noise is reduced, attention returns. It's amazing what a little quiet can do for a child.

As you continue to work with your child and his or her school, stay supportive of teachers' and administrators' efforts on your child's behalf and keep them apprised of the improving results that you see in your child's academic and social abilities. Schools like getting good report cards, too.

Extracurricular Activities

The advocacy you practice in your child's school needs to branch out into every area of interest when a child is dealing with an APD. You need to have an impact on and contribute to creating better listening environments for your child throughout the day and during vacation and summer break as well. Make a list of activities your child participates in during the week. It may include:

- Art classes
- Music lessons
- Dance classes
- Theater
- Academic clubs
- Religious groups
- Girl Scouts and Boy Scouts
- Sports

Reach out to everyone supervising these activities and make sure that they have all the information they need to communicate with your child well and work around any problems that come from his or her APD. Discuss listening differences in very simple and straightforward terms, and explain how APD may affect your child's contributions or performance. Ask for any accommodations your speech-language pathologist recommends and that your child may need.

- Let coaches and instructors know your child may not be able to hear clearly from a distance, especially when directions are yelled from the sidelines or spoken from the back of a room.
- Let your child's coaches know that speaking with your child and the other players before they take the field will get better results than shouting out during the game with performance information that could have been dealt with beforehand.
- Remind coaches to face your child as much as possible so your child can see and hear simultaneously.

Prepare your child for sports and other activities by making what your child is interested in playing or doing as an after-school activity part of the conversations you have and the games the two of you play together. Select age-appropriate books on the sport or topic to read together.

Above all, keep challenging your child and yourself to enjoy everything there is to do, see, and listen to in your world. Don't let APD back your child down from trying something he or she might like. Never let a potentially difficult listening environment dissuade you from giving your child every opportunity to meet the world head-on and enjoy childhood to the fullest. It is not up to us to limit our children's experiences. Our job is to show our sons and daughters how to adapt to the world around them so they have every chance to be happy, have fun, and succeed.

PART THREE

TREATING APD THROUGH SKILL BUILDING

SIX

Strengthening Listening Skills
in the Early Years

Over the course of your child's developmental stages, he will form his own unique canvas of thought processes, ideas, habits, memories, and beliefs based on what he hears, sees, and experiences. The beauty of that creation—how well a child can reason, feel, and participate in the world around him from birth to age five and beyond—depends on how rich his experiences are. The brain builds both from the bottom up and from the top down. Your child's mind will grow based on how much and what kind of information he is given with which to build.

The brain is a remarkable organ—the more quality things it's given to hear, see, feel, and do, the stronger it gets and the deeper it goes. Your child's wide-open, endlessly receptive, miraculously elastic brain needs a steady diet of sounds, images, and experiences that will stretch it, challenge it, and tempt it to go further and deeper. The person who has the most responsibility to see that a child receives those challenges is you, the parent.

Words and language have meaning only when both the speaker and the listener are committed to sharing the process of communication. For children from birth through age five, the bulk of that responsibility rests with the adults who raise them. It's up to mothers, fathers, teachers, and caregivers to ensure that both they and the child they care for are committed to what they're doing together. By working with a child, encouraging him, and narrating activities, a caregiver provides that child with a boost that will be invaluable down the line. What you need to do in order to foster that dual commitment to language and sustain a connection with your child through sound is what's called *joint focus*. Simply making sure that both you and your child pay attention and experience the same object, image, or sound at the same time lays the groundwork for the tasks of conversation, social interaction, and school learning in the future. When both of you participate by jointly focusing and sharing play with toys, taking turns listening and speaking, reading and looking at books, and engaging in other activities and interactions, the stage is set for huge leaps and strides in the child's life ahead.

The following examples demonstrate ways of addressing the six specific auditory processing skills discussed earlier, using activities paired with a story. Using a story gives you and your child a single thing to focus on together and is less stressful and much more fun for you and your child than just doing rote call-and-response exercises. Picture books, especially folk and fairy tales, appeal to children of varying ages.

The words used in these exercises are all found in *The Three Billy Goats Gruff*, a popular children's book adapted from a Norwegian folk tale that is available almost anywhere in several illustrated editions. For the purposes of this group of activities, any version of the book will do, though I like the version by Paul Galdone.

Blake's initial diagnosis revealed that he had difficulty catego-rizing places and things, had word retrieval issues and recall dif-ficulties. Part of his home routine involves our playing a variety of games including Give Me Five, Who Am I?, and Going on a Trip that help Blake with those issues. Give Me Five challenges him to name five of anything in a category (five animals that live in water, five vegetables, five people we know with brown hair) and helps him fine-tune his categorization and recall skills. In Going on a Trip, we talk about what we'll need to pack for travel to a particular location, like Miami (a bathing suit, suntan lotion, a beach blanket). The game Who Am I? is really fun for us. I think of a person he knows and he asks me specific descriptive questions to figure out who I am. "Is it a boy or girl? Does she have brown hair?"—the closer he gets, the more into it he gets. These games are simple yet powerful because they help him have a good time while exercising that unique brain of his.

—ROSIE

IDENTIFICATION

Ask your child to listen for the "s" sound at the end of a word, sig-nifying more than one. A plural can sound three different ways: as an "s," "z," or "es" sound. For this warm-up exercise your child is listening for any of those sounds. All you and your child are try-ing to decide together is whether the word is plural or not. Ask your child to point to the picture in the book that goes with the word that you say.

Sitting next to your child, look at the book together. Say the word "goat" and ask your child to point to what she heard. She should point to one goat. Now say the word "goats." She should point to more than one goat. If your child gets it right, reinforce by saying, "Yes. This is one goat, and these are many goats." If she doesn't get it at first, point to the appropriate picture and say, "Here is one goat; here are many goats. Listen again: goat, goats."

Now try this with other pictures in the book:

flower, flowers
hoof, hooves
river, rivers
troll, trolls
horn, horns
tail, tails

Now have your child listen for the "t" sound at the end of the word. Say the word while your child just listens. You are identifying the ending sound for her or him. "These are words that end in the 't' sound. Listen."

goat	eat	fat	wait
dirt	fruit	rabbit	hat

DISCRIMINATION

In this exercise you are helping your child listen for when words are the same and when they are different. Before saying each pair of words, ask your child, "Are these words the same or different?"

boat, bow (different)

If your child gets it right, reinforce by saying, "Yes, 'bow' and 'boat' are different words." If he misses it, ask your child to listen again. This time give more emphasis to the "t" at the end of "boat" and then say the two words with equal emphasis.

boat, boat (same)

goat, goat (same)

go, goat (different)

eat, ear (different)

eat, eat (same)

weak, wheat (different)

wheat, wheat (same)

SYNTHESIS/SOUND BLENDING

Look at the pictures in the book together. Ask your child, "Tell me the word for what I'm pointing to." Now, do the same activity without the pictures.

You say	*Your child responds*
g-oat	goat
tr-oll	troll
ri-ver	river
t-ai-l	tail
br-i-dge	bridge

AUDITORY CLOSURE

Using a picture at first as a guide and later without a picture

You say	*Response*
"Finish the word for me. The last part is missing. Win_____."	"window"

"Fill in the first part of the word.
_____oll."   "troll"

"Fill in the middle part. fl_____ers"   "flowers"

FOLLOWING DIRECTIONS

Draw or cut out pictures of goats and a troll. Have available crayons, tape, and flat wooden sticks to make stick puppets. (Your child will need to know the words for colors and sizes.)

"Color the big goat red."
"Color the small goat yellow."
"Color the medium-size goat blue."
"Put the yellow goat on the stick."

Continue adding more difficult directions that involve more language.

"Color the biggest goat's horns orange and his beard brown."
"Color the bigger goat's body pink and his tail red."

Just for fun, have your child give you coloring directions. This isn't a listening activity; children love to "be the teacher" and give directions themselves.

FOLLOWING MULTISTEP DIRECTIONS

Create a storyboard together. Ask your child to draw the following:

"On one side of the paper draw a brown hill of dirt."
"On the other side of the paper draw a green hill of grass."

"Between the two draw blue water."
"Over the water draw a bridge from one hill to the other."
"Put the goats on the brown hill."
"Put the troll under the bridge."

AUDITORY MEMORY

Encourage your child to repeat sentences from the story. As she gets the hang of it, increase the length and complexity of the sentence request.

Act out the story using the storyboard you have drawn and the stick puppets you have made. Say a line of dialogue from the book and then ask your child to repeat it and act it out with the puppet: "Who's that walking over my bridge?"

Looking at the parts of the goat (horns, hooves, beard), have your child repeat back these sentences of increasing length, first while looking at the pictures and then listening alone:

"The goat has two horns."
"The goat has two horns on his head."
"The goat has a beard and two horns on his head."
"The big goat has a beard and two horns on his head."
"The biggest goat has a long beard and two horns on his head."

AUDITORY SEQUENTIAL MEMORY

Ask your child to retell the story, first using the pictures from the book, and then without pictures at a later time, like dinner. You might ask your child to "tell Daddy the story we read today," so that he has the opportunity to recall the story events from memory and without any props. Does he remember the story? Are the events of the story in order?

After listening to the story, ask comprehension questions:

"Who are the characters in the story?"
"What is the setting of the story? Where does it take place?"
"The goats have a problem. What is the problem?"
"How do the goats solve the problem?"

In addition to asking questions, you could have a discussion about the story. Be sure to leave room for your child's response by pausing. Sometimes pausing and waiting is the hardest thing to do, but it really does give your child an invitation to discuss his thoughts with you openly. Try using these topic starters:

"That troll was pretty scary." (wait)
"Those goats were very smart." (wait)
"They tricked the troll together." (wait)
"I wonder where the troll went." (wait)

AUDITORY FIGURE/GROUND

Once a child is successful with activities in a quiet setting, you can introduce background noise. Using very light background noise can help desensitize your child to sounds that interfere with her ability to listen in genuinely noisy environments. Introduce instrumental music, then songs with words, and then talking from the radio. Or don't overcontrol natural environmental sounds— for example, keep a window or room door open.

SEVEN

Getting Ready for School: Making the Listening and Learning Connection

Most children are born with the latent capacity to walk. Infants work their way up from waving their hands and feet around to crawling on all fours. With the right encouragement, as their bodies and minds grow, they take their first steps a few at a time, hand in hand with their parents, until eventually they're walking on their own two feet. The same process applies to children's ability to listen. Most kids are also born able to listen. They spend the first year or so of their lives primarily taking in language before beginning to talk in earnest. Through interactions with their family and caregivers, children learn to communicate and reason with increasing confidence and clarity. The learning equivalent of walking on their own two feet comes when they arrive at the first day of kindergarten, usually around age five.

The doorway a child enters when he makes his first trip into the kindergarten classroom is an even more important, far reaching, and challenging transition than the change from crawling to walking. Once a child crosses that threshold, he is ready to take even bigger steps. If everything goes according to plan, he will, with the help of his teachers and shared experiences with his peers, grow into an intellectually and socially capable adult.

Parents wouldn't dream of sending their kids off for their first day of school without a lunch, proper clothing, and books and school supplies. We all struggle to give our children the best preparation possible for the challenges of the important new chapter in our child's life that the first day of school represents. Unfortunately, an increasing number of children arrive for school without one of the single most important things they'll need to succeed—the ability to listen. Whether due to an undiagnosed auditory processing disorder or other problems, every September new students arrive in American schools unable to apply themselves to the central task at hand—learning by listening.

STUDY SKILLS

In American primary school education, there are four different ways of learning. Acquiring, communicating, and exchanging knowledge and experience between teacher and student and from classmate to classmate happens through:

1. Reading
2. Writing
3. Talking
4. Listening

But when we rearrange the same list in order of how much of an average primary school day is devoted to each activity, it actually reads like this:

1. Listening
2. Talking

3. Reading
4. Writing

As much time as kids devote to the three Rs and interacting with each other, children actually spend between 50 percent and 70 percent of each school day learning through listening. It is the single most important skill a child brings with her from home to school. Even though listening is a primary skill that can always be improved, certainly in school-age children, and is one of the first things we begin to learn at birth, it's the form of communication that is taught the least. The actual breakdown looks something like this:

Skill	Order learned at home	Amount used in a school day	Directly taught in school
Listening	First	50% and up	Least
Talking	Second	30% and up	Second least
Reading	Third	16% and up	Second most
Writing	Fourth	9% and up	Most

Why is listening not taught in school? Because educators assume that by the time a child reaches school age she or he will already know how to actively listen. It's up to parents to lay the necessary foundation for a school career of learning by listening. And yet almost every primary school teacher I work with reports that increasingly children arrive for their first school experiences without the auditory skills that they need to succeed.

Ironically, major contributing factors to this lack of basic language and listening skills are the impressive new ways we deliver and share language today. We live in an age where media is everywhere. More than two hundred channels of television, the Internet, video games, text messaging, iPods—these days it feels like we absorb and transmit language from every direction. Television has been condemned as a "vast wasteland" for more than half a century. When it comes to developing listening skills, that's absolutely true. Regardless of an individual parent's stance on violent or offensive TV content, anxiety about TV advertising, politics, values, or age-specific programming, one thing will always keep TV from having a place in a child's formative at-home listening education: television is *passive*. Communication with a TV is one-way only. Children learn listening skills through active application—hearing words, learning their meanings through a variety of contexts, saying those words, and putting them to use. No matter how big your screen is, how high-def the picture or multichannel the audio, children (and adults) don't actively listen to what comes out of the television. They don't need to because nothing is expected of them in return.

Active, engaged listening is an essential part of a child's early development. Watching television during the first few years of life robs kids and parents alike of valuable hours that could be spent giving children quality auditory stimulation, conversation, reading time, playtime, and the active experience of language their hungry growing brains need. The American Academy of Pediatrics has even gone on record saying that until the age of two, children shouldn't watch TV at all. Yet according to a recent study, nearly two-thirds of American kids between birth and age two watch TV regularly. The same study found that one-fifth of our children two and under even have a TV in their bedroom. Half of those kids know how to turn the set on without any help from an adult. This means that a sizable portion of American children have unlimited access to a device that does nothing to contribute to their development and may, merely by

> The first thing that I would say to the parent of a kid with APD or listening issues is turn off the TV and turn off the computer. That's the biggest thing. Just what the commercials alone do to kids who have focus issues—you know, when there are words going by at the bottom of the screen and all this fast talking at different volume levels? It's too fast for kids' brains. You're saying you can't teach your children to focus? Turning off the TV is a start, you know? Read to them every night, have conversations with your kids, and they'll learn to focus better. That's a huge thing. People just don't do it anymore. Parker, Chelsea, Blake, and Vivienne all go to a media-free school and we live together in a media-free house. We have movie night together once a week, but otherwise the TV stays off. And we ask their friends' parents to not let them sit and watch TV instead of playing together. It's not like it's a banned substance or that we're Amish or anything; it's just that Kelli and I don't want the kids to watch TV at someone else's house when we don't do that at home. It's addictive for adults, so imagine what it feels like for kids. They lose themselves in that world.
>
> —ROSIE

the fact that it takes away time that could be spent in healthy interactions with parents and family, be harmful to kids in the long run.

WHAT TO BRING TO SCHOOL

"Education," said Nelson Mandela, "is the most powerful weapon which you can use to change the world." It's true. If we want our kids to wield that all-powerful weapon of education skillfully and responsibly, we must equip them with everything they need to make full use of their school years. Education is communication, and the quickest, simplest, and most direct route to understanding is through listening. We owe it to our kids to give them as much of a head start as we can.

No two children arrive for their first day of school with exactly the same listening skills. Like all of the developmental milestones we examine in this book, the skills and stages described below are based on clinical standards and my own experiences as a speech-language pathologist and a mom. Kindergartners should be able to listen well enough to manage some, if not most or all, of the following classroom activities:

- Know the names of the school subjects they'll be studying, such as math, reading, and the alphabet, and the names of the basic learning tools that they will be using, including scissors, calendar, and eraser
- Know when and how to respond to a teacher's question when called upon, regardless of the answer
- Be able to listen to an age-appropriate story, recall five details from the story and provide basic answers to the "three Ws"—who, what, where
- Recognize what a problem is in a story and that every story problem has a possible solution
- Understand that words are made of component sounds
- Tell whether sounds are the same or different

Again, children's abilities vary, but by first grade ideally a child should:

- Have a solid grasp of phonics—consonants and some vowels, syllables, and the component sounds that form words
- Possess a deeper story understanding that embraces the when, why, and how of age-appropriate literature

- Have an ability to discuss, share, act out, and retell what they've heard
- Show the beginnings of applied rote memorization skills and an ability to repeat things they've learned

All of these activities are based in listening. Whether or not a child grows to school age with an auditory processing disorder to contend with, all children need to step off the school bus the first time armed with an ability to listen. Well-developed childhood listening skills are fed by a generous supply of words. When it comes to giving a child a head start on doing well in the classroom and in social settings, increasing word power is simply priceless.

WORD POWER

From the moment of birth every healthy human being begins a lifelong romance with words and language. An infant may only be able to "say" three or four things that parents recognize after his first six months and won't begin to really use speech to form words until after his twelfth month, but studies show that almost from day one babies meticulously compile a library of the words they repeatedly hear. Adults learn words and use them quickly compared to an infant, toddler, or preschooler. Our grown-up way with words can be so automatic and instantaneous that we mistake the two skills of listening and speaking for the same thing. Many parents and caregivers assume that if a baby can't say many words, the child isn't ready to hear many words. But listening to words and speaking words are two different, complementary skills that become increasingly intertwined as we mature. Listening and speaking each maintain distinct libraries of vocabulary words. The difference is between *receptive vocabulary* (the words we receive, recognize, and understand through listening) and *expressive vocabulary* (the words that we say, share, and communicate through language).

This data bank of known words grows exponentially as a child does.

- From nineteen months to twenty-four months, a child can typically assemble an average receptive vocabulary of some 300+ words.
- Between two and three years, that figure can swell to somewhere between 500 and 900 words.
- From three to four years, when preschool begins, it stretches from 1,200 to 2,000 words on average.
- By four years many children can have more than 2,800 words in their receptive vocabulary.
- From five to six years it increases to an average of 13,000 words.
- And from six to seven years their receptive vocabulary comprises some 20,000 or more words.

A developing infant isn't born ready to use any words, but she is absolutely ready to hear words and begin the process of learning and remembering them and their meanings. As that infant grows to speaking age, her garden of receptive vocabulary needs careful planting, must be fed and added to, tended, cultivated, and admired as it blossoms and flourishes.

PLANTING AND TENDING YOUR CHILD'S WORD GARDEN

Timmy's mother holds her eight-month-old son in her arms as she bends down to safely introduce the child to the neighbors' friendly cocker spaniel. Both boy and canine are curious about the other. "I wonder what that's called," Timmy's mother says to her son before answering herself a suitable pause later. "It's a dog," she says, then again, after a pause, "Dog. That's right, he's a dog." She waits to see if her child imitates the sound of the word she's just said. Then she asks, "Can you say 'dog'?" Enchanted by this friendly, furry creature wagging its tail and by the sound of his mother's voice, Timmy makes an attempt to pronounce the word that's just been offered to him and then giggles. He may not have repeated the word back to his mother, and likely he won't be able to say it clearly for months yet, but already "dog" is on its way to becoming a permanent fixture in Timmy's receptive vocabulary. And the relationship between Timmy and the word that he has heard for the first time is just beginning.

The brain of a growing child is always forging links. Sounds and images, emotions and experiences, tastes and smells—an infant's mental development is a matter of linking new information, feelings, and sensations to old. It's a little like building an elegant palace brick by brick—each new part of the palace is built on a foundation of material that has already been put in place. The relationship between word meaning—the underlying object or concept beneath a spoken or written word label—and the word itself is called *semantics*. The building of vocabulary and the linking of old and new meanings can continue for a lifetime.

We looked earlier at the general numbers of words that children should have in their vocabularies at specific ages. Knowing the meanings of thousands of individual words is vital to a school-age child's academic success and social ease. But word power increases in two ways:

- Vertically—listening and later reading new words that get stacked and stockpiled on top of the ones we already have learned
- Horizontally, by forging new semantic links—additional meanings of words, new words that describe details associ-

ated with those old words, and relationships between new
words and meanings we've already collected

Vocabulary needs to be both a deep well of individual words
and also a broad lake of associations and meanings that distinguish words from each other and link them together for the
fullest possible use in language. Every new word a child learns
can link to additional meanings and uses.

Timmy's initial encounter with the word "dog" came with a
clear, definitive example of what the word means. The semantic
context Timmy first has for "dog" is the wagging, friendly creature that lives at his neighbors' house. As Timmy is exposed to
more examples of dogs—experiences where he listens to the
word being spoken and links new information specific to that
event with the old context—the word "dog" will grow horizontally in his mind. The neighbors' dog is a cocker spaniel. The next
dog Timmy encounters may be a Great Dane, a beagle, or a poo-
dle. Timmy won't learn these words for some time yet, but he will
recognize that there are more ways of understanding and communicating about dogs and what makes them similar and different from one another. As he gets older, Timmy's mind will
broaden the meaning of "dog" by using the word as a category for
animals that, like his neighbors' cocker spaniel, have defining details such as fur, four legs, paws, floppy or pointy ears, and a tail;
pants and barks; and come when they're called by name. That
category will naturally split and subdivide and details will create
more connections as Timmy's experience with the word "dog"
grows and his ability to use words deepens. Multiple meanings of
"dog" make his understanding even richer: a stuffed animal with
many of the same physical details as the real thing or a picture
book about a cartoon animal that looks like a dog but acts human
helps Timmy vertically stack useful words that categorize, describe, and distinguish these various dogs both from real dogs

Timmy has met and from each other. At the same time Timmy's semantic understanding of just what a dog is expands horizontally. Once he enters school, starts using language more, and continues to listen, the semantic meaning of "dog" grows along with him—as a metaphoric turn of phrase, idiom, slang, and so on.

When a child struggles with listening difficulties, developmental problems, or an auditory processing disorder, both vertical and horizontal word growth are at risk. Unable to listen to each word spoken to him or her and ill-equipped to focus on and remember multiple words and multiple meanings, the kid with APD wrestles with the growing demands of vocabulary—so much so that many parents fail to challenge their child with APD to increase his individual word power. If Timmy's mother heard her son say the word "dog" and use it as a label for what they were looking at together, she may feel justified in not wanting to challenge her son any further. Parents will often let their child with APD fall back on either using a single general word to cover multiple semantic meanings that call for words of their own, or allow the child to retain a simplistic definition of a word with multiple meanings and potential uses in language. This sets up the child for a difficult time once he enters school. It's not unreasonable to expect a child to eventually know that "puppy" is a word for a baby dog, for example, and for parents to bring other dog-related words such as "canine," "pooch," and "mutt" into the mix. In my practice, when I hear kids using words such as "stuff," "things," or "you know what I mean" to describe a broad variety of different objects or ideas they should know the real names of, it's clear that there's work to be done.

WORD POWER BOOST

When playing and spending time with your child, be mindful of the opportunity to use this time to help her build the two axes of vocabulary. Take the example "ship." A two-year-old might have a toy ship, or you might point one out on a trip or vacation. The two of you could encounter the picture of a ship in a book you read together, or an older child might see one in a book she is reading. A good technique is to take a word such as "ship," encountered during playtime, together time, or story time, and use it to extend vocabulary both vertically and horizontally using *categories, descriptions, multiple meanings, synonyms,* and *antonyms.*

Categories

Establish that your child has said the word "ship" and not "sip" or something else that sounds similar. Then ask him questions that will sort "ship" into groups of other words.

> Things that are big like ships: dinosaur, school building, bridge . . .
> Things people ride in: airplane, car, bus, spaceship . . .
> Things made of wood: house, baseball bat, tree . . .
> Things made of metal: bike, tin can, frying pan . . .
> Kinds of ships: submarine, sailing ship, pirate ship . . .
> Objects that you find at the ocean: fish, lighthouse, seal, penguin . . .

Work out subcategories that branch out associations from "ship."

> Places you see ships: in oceans, in books, on rivers, on lakes . . .
> People you find on ships: sailors, a captain, pirates . . .
> Things on board a ship: sails, cannons, ropes . . .

Descriptions

Each one of these words comes with words that describe it and its relation to "ship." Explore those details together. For example, you could say, "A dinosaur can be as big as a ship. Some are small, too."

Encourage your child to use or learn descriptive words to make connections: "You can ride on a ship. Could you ride on a dinosaur?"

Multiple Meanings

"Ship" can mean "boat" or it can mean "send for delivery." The word "ship" is in common phrases such as "shipshape" and "ship ahoy." Discuss some of these word alternatives and overlaps with your child.

Synonyms

Help your child discover and explore other words that mean the same or nearly the same as "ship."

As a noun: boat, craft, vessel . . .
As a verb: send, mail, transport . . .

Antonyms

Play with words or concepts that mean the opposite of "ship." With concrete nouns such as "ship" we can broaden the definition of antonym to include objects that do some of the same things as ships do but aren't the same as ships, or situations where a ship no longer works in the ways you've already discussed.

Similar function: airplane, bus, house . . .
No longer works like a ship: shipwreck, sinking ship . . .

Making a habit of helping your child collect more vocabulary words and create links between words in this way is a great system for increasing your child's word power. Using your time together to expand and grow vocabulary is a good way for the two of you to interact, communicate, and learn how each other's mind works. Sharing language is connecting. Of course, it's impossible to do this each time the two of you see something together. Not every interaction needs to be a lesson—but every lesson is an opportunity to connect.

RULES OF THE ROAD FOR SCHOOL SUCCESS

Children have a capacity for observation and imitation that's simply amazing. It's a skill that they use in order to learn, grow, and develop into increasingly mature people able to deal with tasks and experiences of increasing complexity. They're watching us and they're listening to us, so it's important for us to model good listening and communication skills for them.

- Get down to your child's level while talking.
- Give your child your full attention when she speaks.
- Make eye contact and demonstrate with your expression that you are interested in what your child has to say.
- Listen patiently—children think faster than they can speak. With limited vocabulary and experience in talking, children often take longer than adults to find the right word.
- Try not to interrupt your child before she has finished speaking.
- Remember that children return the respect they receive. Children who have been listened to tend to become good listeners themselves.
- Get in the habit of giving your child simple instructions. Start with one-step directions such as "Bring me your sweater" or "Hold up the book." As your child becomes a

more sophisticated listener, you can add another task or two, such as "Pick up that toy down the hall and put it in your room," and eventually three-step directions, such as "Put your shoes on, get your coloring book, and hop in the car."

TEACH SUCCESS

Remember that you're not testing your child; you're helping him to fulfill his potential and to fully experience his world. Using "I" messages is a powerful way of letting your child know he has been successful: "I like the way you listened to the story" or "I think what you said is so interesting." These statements personalize praise and approval.

There are so many other words and phrases we can use to praise our children. Encourage your child with:

wow	well done	excellent	bravo
great job	fantastic	nice work	beautiful
spectacular	magnificent	sensational	outstanding
terrific	wonderful	awesome	phenomenal
congratulations			

Use expressions like:

I am so proud of you	I knew you could do it
You are incredible	Now you've got it
Much better	You are so clever
I am so impressed	You figured it out
You are so creative	I like the way you listen
You are so thoughtful	You are such a joy

We all like to be praised for something well done, but excessive praise dilutes the effect. Make sure your approval and the words you choose to express it are authentic. Positive reinforcement works when you "catch" your child doing good. Point out when your child does or says something particularly positive, kind, or imaginative over the course of the day, not just when you are engaged in teaching time.

Don't forget, no matter what happens, that a big hug, a kiss, and a warm smile communicate volumes about how you feel.

INTEGRATION

Of course, the competing demands of your career, your marriage, the needs of your other children, and the dozens of other responsibilities you juggle don't just go away because one child has an auditory processing disorder or needs additional attention in the years leading up to kindergarten. The way to make the most of your time and your child's time is to strike a balance. You don't need to constantly stimulate and verbally engage your child all day long; just try to make the most of the time you do spend with him or her. Find fifteen minutes each day that you can share with your child in which you can work on listening skills. The key to helping your son or daughter acquire the tools he or she needs to arrive prepared for the first day of school is *integration*—successfully blending the practicing and sharpening of listening skills with the daily activities you do anyway. Using everyday activities to help grow your daughter or son's listening skills also gives your child a familiar and reassuring background of everyday situations to build on, as well as a comforting one-on-one dynamic that won't cause your child to feel pressured or scrutinized.

During the first year of life your child is listening and gaining information. In the example Timmy learned the word "dog" and then added more words that link in meaning and association at greater and greater levels of sophistication and complexity. "Dog" brings "big dog" and then, as Timmy gets older, "I see a big dog," "That big dog is funny," and so on. By the time your child reaches age two, he or she has already benefited from the examples you've set and the information you've shared by talking to your child, narrating the activities you perform together, asking simple questions, and giving your child useful answers to think about and remember.

The ideas below are suggestions and examples, not a script to be followed. Think about the activities you share with your child as chances to use your imagination and build upon the scenarios and age-appropriate developmental tips below. You know your daughter or son better than anyone, and with some practice, patience, and love, you should get a sense of what works well as he or she grows and you go about your daily routine.

Age Two: Mealtime

Being able to point at objects with your child and give them a word label is the best way to share and grow vocabulary in a two-year-old. Preparing food, eating, and washing up after meals offer lots of opportunities to make those word connections together.

- Point to and identify food ingredients and cooking implements using the objects themselves and the pictures and words on can labels and cereal boxes.
- Add adjectives to the nouns you indicate. Describe food as "spicy," "hot," "cold," "soft," and so on. Cereal can be "crunchy cereal."

- Use verbs both with the names of foods and with the descriptive adjectives: "pouring cereal," "pouring crunchy cereal."
- Explore numbers and plurals together—count spoons and cups as you set or clear the table. Share the distinction between "plate" and "plates."
- Play different kinds of music at lunch and talk to your child about whether he likes it or not and why.

Age Three: Grocery Store

We want to continue expanding our three-year-old child's vocabulary, adding words that may not be in her immediate environment and helping her to name things she discovers for herself. Three-year-olds are ready to group words together into categories. The supermarket is a great place to explore word categories ("vegetables," "fruits," "meats," etc.), add new adjectives and antonyms ("heavy" versus "light," "smooth" versus "rough," "raw" versus "cooked," etc.) and new verbs ("weigh," "freeze," "stack"), and use numbers, colors, and shapes for descriptions.

- Name the fruits and vegetables you see (whether your child eats them or not).
- Weigh them on a scale and call out the numbers.
- Talk about the colors, shapes, and sizes of foods and how they compare.
- Discuss quantities of foods—"gallon," "pound," "can," "box," "bunch," "dozen," and so on.
- Talk about the foods you like and those you don't.
- Explore the words for the parts of the supermarket— "checkout counter," "cash register," "dairy case."
- Select fruit together, bring it home, and talk about what you are doing as you make a fruit salad and eat it together.

Age Four: Farm

A four-year-old can add even more word categories and fill in more details to describe what you see. More description adds more words and expands a child's perspective.

- Talk about the animals. "Where do they live?" "What do they eat?" "What do they give us or do?" "Hens give us eggs, cows give us milk, we ride horses."
- Describe what they look like and compare them to other animals, such as zoo animals or pets at home. What is the same? What is different?
- Make as many subcategories as you can out of farm animals—animals with four legs, animals with two legs, animals with horns, animals with fur, animals with feathers, baby animals, animals that are bigger than a child, animals that are smaller than a child, animals that make sounds. Talk about how the categories overlap—a chicken has two legs and feathers, makes sounds, and is smaller than a child.
- Explore the similarities and differences between words in a category—"dog" and "hog," "cow" and "crow," and so on.

Age Five: Aquarium

By age five your child will probably be ready to discuss and describe word categories in even more detail. Examining the how, what, when, where, and why of the things the two of you look at and talk about together will help to build word power and extend vocabulary and meaning.

- Describe fish by color or size using more specific words and phrases, such as "blue-green" or "the size of your hand."

A POST OFFICE TRIP

A trip to the post office offers different variations as a language and vocabulary opportunity for children of different ages.

One-Year-Old: Nouns and Verbs

Talk about the noun and the action.

> "I have a letter."
> "Let's mail the letter."
> "There's the mailbox."
> "Let's put it in the mailbox."
> "There it goes."
> "Great—all done!"

Two-Year-Old: Adding Activity and Destination

Do a simple action together before going to the post office and link what you are doing with where you are going.

> "Let's write a letter to Grandma."
> "Can you color a picture?"
> "Let's put it in an envelope."
> "We'll mail it to Grandma at the post office."
> "Put the letter in the mailbox."

Three-Year-Old: Asking Questions

Let your child make choices and decisions about your activities.

> "Whom should we write to?"
> "What should we say? You tell me and I will write it. Dear Grandma . . ."

"Can you write your name?" (Your child may just make marks on the paper.)

"Let's put it in an envelope."

"We'll go to the post office."

"Where should we put the letter?"

Four-Year-Old: More Options

A four-year-old child is ready for more choices.

"Whom should we write to?"

"What should we write? Can you help me? Draw the picture and tell me what to write."

"We need an envelope and a stamp."

"Who will deliver this letter? . . . The mail carrier?"

"Let's go to the post office."

"We need Grandma's address."

"Where does she live? In Connecticut? Is that far away?"

Five-Year-Old: Taking Charge

A five-year-old will want to lead an activity and perform more independently. The child also can use her powers of predication.

"Whom should we write to?"

"You can write to Grandma."

"Do you need help spelling? I'll tell you the letters—you write."

"That's great—now how are we going to mail this?"

"What should we do first? . . . Next? . . . And last?"

"Great! I wonder when Grandma will get the letter."

- Compare and contrast fish using distinctive features: "sharp teeth," "small eyes," "slow-moving."
- How are they the same? How are they different? Which ones do people eat? What bodies of water do they swim in? What part of the world do they come from? Are they dangerous? Why or why not?
- Ask and answer questions to stimulate conversation. Try using "I wonder . . ." ("I wonder what that fish eats," "I wonder how that fish moves so quickly") and "Maybe . . ." ("Maybe it eats little fish," "Maybe it's a very strong swimmer").

Mealtimes, the supermarket, trips to the playground, cleaning or doing the laundry, bath time, getting ready for school, errands, going to the library, visits to a zoo or farm or aquarium, an afternoon at a museum, traveling to another city to visit relatives—at any age these are center-stage locations and activities for helping your children boost their word power and prepare for the school-age world around the corner.

to listening, there's a specific division of labor within the organ that houses our minds. The left side of the brain deals with language and the vocabulary and logic behind it. At the same time, the right side handles the rhythm, intonation, and patterns of language—what's known in clinical circles as *prosody*. The human mind does its best work when both sides of the brain communicate freely and harmoniously to make sense of and enjoy the constantly changing kaleidoscope of experience. The real magic of listening, thinking, and doing happens when the right and left brain take on the world as one.

Music and musical language encourage both sides of a child's mind to happily get to work. When a child listens to and learns simple rhymes and song patterns, left-brain functions such as vocabulary and grammar join up with right-brain functions such as prosody, feeling, and intuition. When it comes to listening and language development, that two-sided brain "conversation" is simply crucial. Music engages the left and right auditory processing centers fully. It encourages a deepening relationship between sound, memory, and movement, and strengthens a child's capacity to communicate and reason effectively. All kinds of separate brain functions come together as repeated beats, rhymes, and sound patterns create new pathways and new connections on both sides of a child's growing mind.

For hundreds, probably thousands, of years, just about every culture on earth has used a music-like form of expression to help their children grow supple minds that freely exchange information, ideas, and sensations between both sides of the brain. Like a song, a nursery rhyme combines tempo, tone, and rhythm into a potent language cocktail perfectly suited to a developing child's listening and learning needs.

Nursery rhymes have been passed down from parent to child for generations. They are one of the oldest, most reliable, and

EIGHT

Music to the Ears: Using Rhythm and Rhyme to Build Listening Skills

The effect that musical sounds and rhythms have on children can be nothing short of miraculous. The words, melody, and tempo of a favorite song can turn a shy child into a giggling, squealing dervish, or calm and relax a child who's running wild. Listening to musical sounds has incredible long-term benefits, too. The beats, notes, and words making up even the simplest song are a feast of healthily complex auditory information and sensation for your child's stimulation-hungry growing brain. Music and music-like recitations, such as poems and chants, don't just entertain and strengthen young minds; they actually encourage the two halves of the brain to talk to each other. What a boon this can be to the child with an APD!

You've seen pictures showing the distinctive cleft through the center of human gray matter marking a division between the two sides, or hemispheres, of the brain. And you've probably also heard or read about the brain's two-sided nature. When it comes

I can honestly say that music has been instrumental in helping Blake and me have meaningful exchanges about his feelings. Blake really enjoys music and constantly asks me what the lyrics to particular songs mean. When lyrics to a song he likes use figurative or metaphoric language and have a lot of images in them, that can lead to a conversation about the merging of art, feeling, and fact. "I get knocked down but I get up again" is part of the chorus to a song that Blake loves. "Is that about a football player, Mom?" he'll ask me, or "Is that about boxing?" I'll tell him that, yes, it could be about a sports player and then point out that it could also be about how sometimes even when we feel sad, helpless, or defeated, we still need to have the courage to try working on something that matters to us. These conversations help him describe his frustrations with communication and the difficulties he faces within his sibling relationships, and they give me an opportunity to check in with him and make suggestions about how we can try to make things better even when that's hard to do. The great thing is that the songs and lyrics open up the lines of communication between us and give us an opportunity to share low-stress teachable moments about things that don't come easily to him.

—ROSIE

easiest-to-use teaching tools. They have deep roots in every global culture and help link our children to the past while preparing them for the future. Traditions of any kind come with a use-them-or-lose-them condition attached. The potential for learning and for connecting parents and children that is contained in a simple nursery rhyme is so unique and powerful that to lose that tradition would be a terrible, terrible waste.

THE POWER OF NURSERY RHYMES

There are a number of things that make nursery rhymes one of the best teaching tools for parents to share with children of all listening abilities, but especially those with APD:

- Babies and young children need to learn how to focus and practice paying attention. Children can practice learning to listen for sounds and attend to their sources through familiar rhymes.
- Listening to and learning nursery rhymes encourages children to develop an interest in and curiosity about language.
- Rhyming is engaging and fun. Nursery rhymes give children word sounds they'll remember, want to imitate, and naturally put into the right sequence. The similarities and differences between words stand out in a nursery rhyme. That contrast helps children understand the variety and rich musicality of the sounds, beats, and patterns that make up language. Learning nursery rhymes also gives a child a way to practice fluent, intelligible speech.
- Being taught nursery rhymes accustoms your developing child to the sharing, listening, and repeating that are the foundation of conversation. Rhymes help children to practice the social side of listening to and speaking with another person.
- Repetition and memorization are two of the vital keys to learning. Nursery rhymes are based on repeating and remembering sounds, beats, and words.
- Rhythm and rhyme encourage moving, seeing, and touching, adding a rich multisensory dimension to learning.
- The social connection and safe invitation to interact that parents extend to their children through rhymes becomes the blueprint for the way children relate to their peers. The

Do you remember some of these classic rhymes?

I'm a Little Teapot

I'm a little teapot, short and stout
Here is my handle, here is my spout . . .

Twinkle, Twinkle, Little Star

Twinkle, twinkle, little star
How I wonder what you are . . .

The Mockingbird

Hush little baby, don't say a word
Mama's gonna buy you a mockingbird . . .

same nursery rhymes taught to different children provide a common experience kids can use to bond and connect with each other.

- As your child grows older and the nursery rhymes he learns become more complex, rhyming teaches your child new vocabulary and expressions and contributes to more sophisticated reading and spelling skills.

- It's easy to incorporate nursery rhymes into your and your child's daily life and routine. They're free and can be done anywhere.

- Nursery rhymes help children laugh about things that can be scary or stressful. The fact that the often old-fashioned, exaggerated images and situations in a nursery rhyme are repeated over and over puts a safe, silly, familiar face on primal fears and anxieties such as falling down, getting lost, losing things, being frightened by spiders and other creatures, and so forth.

- Nursery rhymes help you to be patient and respectful of a child's abilities and attentions. When you rhyme together, you are listening to each other. Nursery rhymes connect your child to you.
- Learning, memorizing, repeating, and exchanging rhymes touches on nearly every aspect of listening that may be affected by APD. Children with auditory processing difficulties stand to gain the most by working on rhythm, memory, and accuracy through rhyming games.

LEARNING TO RHYME

Children learn how to rhyme through listening. They get better and better at it by interacting with you. The initially one-way and later two-way listening that nursery rhymes require is a skill and ongoing process that evolves over time. The first step to teaching rhymes is to model the rhyme. Speak the rhyme clearly at a tempo and an emphasis that engages you; this will engage your young child as well. Repeating the rhyme at different times and with different emphases will make what you say familiar and welcome to hear. You can teach a child of speaking age who has heard you recite and perform the rhyme several times how to do it herself in a few easy steps and by remembering a few simple rules.

- Begin by inviting your child to repeat each of the lines after you.
- Speak slowly at first. Children need time to process and to understand the words you say.
- Many nursery rhymes have or suggest movements that go with the rhythm. Teach your child the moves that go with a rhyme by gently holding her hands or moving her arms

Here are some more classic rhymes you can perform for your
infant or teach your toddler:

"Little Miss Muffet"
"Humpty Dumpty"
"To Market, to Market"
"Ring Around the Rosy"
"London Bridge"
"Pease Porridge Hot"
"Hot Cross Buns"

and legs in tune with the lyrics. As your child becomes
more familiar with the movements, ask her to imitate the
motions you make. You can do this with infant children,
too, by taking them in your arms and gently rocking, swaying, or bouncing them to the beat of the rhyme.

- As the rhyme starts to click for your child, try pausing ex-
pectantly in the middle of a phrase and give her a chance to
say the words and perform the movements on her own.

- Praise your child's efforts while you sing the rhyme. Laugh
and play together.

- Don't be afraid to act silly. Nursery rhymes may seem non-
sensical from an adult perspective, but children don't need
the words to make conventional sense.

- Remember that children need to hear nursery rhymes over
and over again before they connect with them enough to
say them on their own. You may tire of the repetition, but
your child craves it. Repetition, familiarity, and safety are
tightly allied in a child's mind. Be patient and willing and
give your child plenty of opportunities to hear, practice, and
use the rhymes you share.

ENRICHING RHYMING TIME

Our kids naturally do their best work when activities and experiences engage several of their senses at once, and this is particularly true for children who are struggling with auditory processing. Anything you can do to bring rhymes to life and increase what your child sees, feels, and hears as you rhyme together will make rhyming time quality time. There are many creative ways to make the experience of rhyming deeper and more useful for your child's development. The simplest and most effective way to add more to rhyming is to emphasize the beats of a rhyme. Adding a physical component to what your child listens to encourages him to experience language with his whole body, not just his ears.

Try clapping out the beats of a nursery rhyme. Clapping the beat helps children develop an awareness of the sounds and individual syllables that make up words. When a child can identify syllables, he's on his way to learning to read and spell. Go slowly through this nursery rhyme and gently clap out the syllable beats, making sure that your child can see your hands coming together and apart.

Hickory Dickory Dock
Hick-o-ry dick-o-ry dock
The mouse ran up the clock
The clock struck one
The mouse ran down
Hick-o-ry dick-o-ry dock

Clapping to mark the beat this way is especially important for children with APD and other listening disorders. Children with auditory processing disorder often struggle to distinguish different syllables. They have a harder time learning vocabulary and using language as a result. A child with APD can learn to use rhymes better if he experiences rhythm in a tactile way, feeling the pieces that make up a word. You can clap, or you can lightly and playfully tap a finger or pencil on a tabletop or on your child's arm or leg in time with the syllable beats.

Another way to enrich the experience of rhythm and rhyme is to use a felt board. Most educational toy stores and retail websites that cater to very young children's needs sell felt boards and a variety of colorful felt pieces in the shape of objects, animals, and characters for $15 or less. You can easily and cheaply buy the materials to make one of your own at a craft store, too. Use the felt board characters and shapes to act out, illustrate, and add personality and color to the words of the rhymes you share. It's also fun for your child if you cut out custom felt character shapes from their favorite rhymes.

Finger puppets offer a wonderful way to extend the enjoyment and power of rhymes. When you perform with finger puppets, it makes the rhyme into an interactive show your child will enjoy while learning. When your child wears the puppets, it makes a nursery rhyme a show he enjoys presenting to you while he increases his dexterity.

RHYMING VARIATIONS

Remember, language is the key to getting the most out of social situations. Children need to practice hearing the emotional shading we use to express our feelings when we interact with each other socially. Most children respond to these changes naturally. When you sound happy and excited, they respond by becoming happy and excited. But children fine-tune their understanding of emphases over time by listening and imitating. Children with APD can be particularly unsure of the meanings and emotional shadings from inflections and emphasis. Over time they can become withdrawn in social situations because they haven't laid the groundwork for understanding different intonations and emphases. It particularly helps them to establish these skills and improve them as they grow when you practice changing the intonation of your voice as you recite nursery rhymes. As you rhyme for an infant or with a toddler, try making your voice louder and softer, higher and lower. You can emphasize the words that rhyme:

The Itsy-Bitsy Spider
*The **itsy-bitsy** spider went up the water **spout***
*Down **came** the **rain** and washed the spider **out***
Out** came the sun and dried up all the **rain
*The **itsy-bitsy** spider went up the spout **again***

Or stress different phrases:

*The itsy-bitsy spider went **up the water spout***
*Down came the rain and **washed the spider out***
*Out came the sun and **dried up all the rain***
*The itsy-bitsy spider **went up the spout again***

Recite a familiar nursery rhyme, emphasizing words that start with the same sound and tapping out each syllable of the rhyme on a tabletop.

Jack and Jill
***Jack** and **Jill** went up the hill*
To fetch a pail of water
***Jack** fell down and broke his crown*
*And **Jill** came tumbling after*

Ask your child to think of other words that start with the letter "J."

A GARDEN OF RHYMES

There are literally hundreds of terrific nursery rhymes to choose from. The full range of Mother Goose and other rhyming books for every age are available at any public library. I also recommend the CD *Humpty Who? A Crash Course in 80 Nursery Rhymes for Clueless Moms and Dads* by Jennifer Griffin. The disc comes with a complete book of the text of the rhymes so you can read along. Spend time playing the CD while you are in the car running errands or at home preparing meals. Hearing the familiar rhymes will help your child visualize the pictures and illustrations she knows from reading together or from felt board and finger puppets activity.

If your child seems engaged and rhymes well, say the first part of the rhyme and ask your daughter or son to finish it: "Jack and Jill went up the _____." Next, you can ask your child, "I wonder what else rhymes with 'Jill.' Does 'pool' rhyme with 'Jill'? 'Jill' and 'pool' . . . no. How about 'pill'? 'Jill' and 'pill'—yes! What else rhymes with 'Jill'?"

Every time you repeat a nursery rhyme you have an opportunity to add or change a dimension of listening, add new layers of meaning, and give your child something new to learn and enjoy.

RHYMING AND SPEAKING

You can use rhymes to teach children to articulate and speak sounds more clearly. When adults go from making a "d" sound to an "f" sound, we quickly, skillfully, and more or less unconsciously change the position of our teeth, tongue, and lips. A growing child may not find that so easy at first. Nursery rhymes can help kids practice skillful, accurate pronunciation. The repetitive sequences in nursery rhymes allow our kids to practice the kind of mouth shapes and movements they will use to speak.

Hey Diddle Diddle
Hey diddle, diddle
The cat and the fiddle
The cow jumped over the moon
The little dog laughed to see such sport
And the dish ran away with the spoon

Nursery rhymes expose children to sounds that may be hard for them to pronounce. "R" is a difficult sound that children sometimes don't successfully master till age six or older. Rhymes that contain the letter "r" in a variety of short and multisyllable words can give children lots of exercise saying this sound.

Row, Row, Row Your Boat
Row, row, row your boat
Gently down the stream
Merrily, merrily, merrily, merrily
Life is but a dream

Working on pronunciation with rhymes is a wonderful, low-stress way to teach your child in a fun, playful, and naturally relaxed way. Instead of focusing on what he is doing wrong, you are giving him lots of practice on how to say it right.

RHYMING AND SEQUENTIAL MEMORY

As we've already seen, the principle of remembering and duplicating word order in language can be extremely difficult to master, especially for a child with an auditory processing disorder.

Nursery rhymes teach children to listen, think, and remember their way through a word sound by sound and through a sentence word by word. The rhythm and repetition make it easy for children to remember the order of the words. Rhymes and songs about the alphabet, ordinal numbers, and months of the year are particularly effective in reinforcing your child's skill with auditory sequential memory.

A B C D E F G
H I J K L M N O P
Q R S, T U V
W X, Y and Z
Now I know my ABCs
Next time won't you sing with me?

One, two, buckle my shoe
Three, four, shut the door
Five, six, pick up sticks
Seven, eight, lay them straight
Nine, ten, do it again

Thirty days hath September
April, June, and November
February has twenty-eight alone
All the rest have thirty-one
Excepting leap year, that's the time
When February's days are twenty-nine

FROM RHYMING TO READING

Children must be aware of the relationship between sounds and symbols before they can learn how to read. The ability to read is a journey of understanding how sounds indicate letters, letters combine to make syllables, syllables combine to make words, and words combine to make sentences. Right from the start of a child's listening life, nursery rhymes can help to lay a strong foundation for reading and spelling by teaching her how to hear, discriminate, store, and retrieve sounds.

Recognizing when one sound ends and another sound begins is a skill that needs to be learned. Mastering how to discriminate between speech sounds takes years of practice. Nursery rhymes can help. The repetition of nursery rhymes teaches children to use *phonemes*—the smallest individual units of sound that we recognize as language and join to make words. Look at and listen to the following rhyme:

Baa Baa Black Sheep
Baa baa black sheep, have you any wool?
Yes sir, yes sir, three bags full
One for the master, one for the dame
And one for the little boy who lives down the lane

Recite the rhyme a few times to your child, clapping or tapping for emphasis if need be. Now recite it again, but pause after "Baa baa black sheep" and point out the "b" sound to your child. "Oh, listen . . . That sound—'baa baa black,' 'b,' 'b,' 'b'—I wonder what that sound is?" Then either point out or draw the letter "b" on a piece of paper and explain, "It's 'b,' the letter 'b'!"

This simple technique can be done with virtually any nursery rhyme to begin translating what your child hears into written words she will eventually read.

A collection of Mother Goose rhymes will introduce your child to the concept of storytelling and help her to be a lifelong lover of books and reading. Starting a child's journey to reading with nursery rhymes also teaches her about the wonders she'll find ahead in books. A rhyme is like a book in miniature—a short little story that can be silly, funny, or scary, and stir a child's imagination while the rhythm holds her attention. As your child learns to listen for the beginning, middle, and ending of the story, she begins to anticipate and imagine what comes next. Being able to predict or wonder about a sequence of events and what happens next is an important step in understanding the plot of the longer stories your child will encounter later. Rhyming introduces your child to concepts of storytelling and narrative, sets the stage for the kind of imaginative curiosity that only books can satisfy, and raises the curtain on a lifelong love of reading.

AGES AND STAGES

Nursery rhymes can help your child learn how to listen more effectively during every stage of growth and development. The rhymes children hear as infants, learn as toddlers, and use as the basis for speaking, listening, and reading in their preteen years will stay with them forever.

Birth to One Year

In their first year, children learn to explore the musicality of language through nursery rhymes. It does not matter if they are too young to understand the meaning of words. Connect the tempo and meter of the rhymes you recite to your little one by swaying, rocking, or gently bouncing her or him as you sing to them. Babies enjoy listening to the rhythmic sounds of nursery rhymes and lullabies while getting gently bounced to the beat or rocked to the rhythm of a song.

Remember, you are not looking for a specific response from your child yet. And an infant will never judge the quality of your voice. It makes no difference if you sing or speak well or if you are even able to carry a tune.

You can begin to play rhyming games with your baby by patting his hands together as you say:

Patty cake, patty cake, baker's man
Bake me a cake as fast as you can
Pat it, prick it and mark it with a "B"
And put it in the oven for baby and me

It's a good idea to start narrating activities as you move through the day. Make up little songs about getting dressed, eating, or bathing.

This is the way we wash our hands, wash our hands, wash our hands
This is the way we wash our toes, wash our toes, wash our toes
This is the way we wash our nose, wash our nose, and wash our nose

Birth to One Year: Books
During the first year, books are of course only read to your infant. These book suggestions all use simple rhythms, easy rhymes, and basic sounds and have large, colorful illustrations so that you can expose your baby to the ritual of reading.

Animal Crackers: A Delectable Collection of Pictures, Poems, Songs and Lullabies for the Very Young by Jane Dyer
Mama, Mama by Jean Marzollo
Hush Kitten by Emanuel Schongut
The Me I See by Barbara Shook Hazen
Say Goodnight by Helen Oxenbury

One to Two Years

As toddlers learn to stand on their own, they are ready for rhymes that help them learn about their bodies. Teach this rhyme by first pointing out the appropriate part of the body on yourself and then on your child:

Why don't you do the head and shoulders with me?
Head, shoulders, knees and toes, knees and toes,
Eyes and ears and mouth and nose . . .

One to Two Years: Books

These book suggestions have more text, more challenging vocabulary and sounds, and more variety in subject matter.

Humpty Dumpty and Other Rhymes by Rosemary Wells
Time for Bed by Mem Fox
Five Little Monkeys Jumping on the Bed by Eileen Christelow
Moo, Baa, La La La by Sandra Boynton
Wake Up, Big Barn by Suzanne Tanner Chitwood
Henny-Penny by Jane Wattenburg

Three to Four Years

Preschoolers can remember only a few words at a time. Their ability to memorize is still developing and they like short, simple rhymes about familiar toys and activities. Continue to narrate experiences for your child as you do chores around the house. You can use the tune from "Here We Go Round the Mulberry Bush" and make up your own lyrics.

Here we go round the mulberry bush, the mulberry bush,
    the mulberry bush
Here we go round the mulberry bush, so early in the morning

This is the way we make the bed, make the bed, make the bed
This is the way we make the bed, so early Monday morning

This is the way we put on your shirt, put on your shirt, put on your
   shirt
This is the way we put on your shirt, so early Tuesday morning

Songs like this teach musical skills and help your child to become creative with language.

Do this next rhyme where you have enough space to act out the jumping motion for your child.

Jack be nimble, Jack be quick
Jack jump over the candle stick
Jack jumped high, Jack jumped low
Jack jumped over and burned his toe

Emphasizing words that rhyme works well with preschoolers. Ask your child if she can hear which sounds are similar and different: "Jack jumped low and burned his toe. Oh, listen, 'low' and 'toe'—they sound alike. I wonder what other words sound like 'toe.' Does 'shoe' sound the same as 'toe'? 'Shoe' and 'toe' . . . no, they sound different. How about 'snow'? 'Snow' and 'toe' . . . yes, they sound alike."

Preschoolers love to practice integrating movement and music in a rhyme like "The Wheels on the Bus." Move your hands in a circular motion as you recite the first verse of this rhyme:

The wheels on the bus go round and round, round and round, round
   and round
The wheels on the bus go round and round, all through the town

Now swish your hands in front of you like a windshield wiper:

*The wipers on the bus go swish swish swish, swish swish swish, swish
swish swish*
The wipers on the bus go swish swish swish, all through the town

Also, nursery rhymes can be a great bridge when children this age and older have difficulty transitioning quickly and smoothly from one activity to another. Reciting a nursery rhyme will engage your child's attention and keep her busy as you move from one task to the next. This comes in especially handy when it's time to stop playing or doing something your child likes to do and start in with something she would rather not do.

Tell your child what's going to happen next and then invite her to end one activity and participate in a new one. For example: "It is time to wash your hands and have lunch now. Would you like to help me do a rhyme while we put away your toys?"

Remember, preschool children have a short attention span, so let your child's interest be your guide. Don't urge her to continue singing or doing nursery rhymes if she's stopped paying attention.

Three to Four Years: Books

These recommended books are more complex. There's more humor and more suggestions of empathy and sympathy for characters. Reading time can be more interactive now. Stop and ask questions of your child and encourage him to rhyme on his own based on the rhymes in the book.

Brown Bear, Brown Bear, What Do You See? by Bill Morton, Jr.
When Mama Comes Home Tonight by Eileen Spinelli
Green Eggs and Ham by Dr. Seuss
Where's My Teddy? by Jez Alborough

Four to Five Years

Children love to sing at this stage of development. They're especially drawn to interactive play songs, such as "Bingo" and "If You're Happy and You Know It," that allow them to participate by clapping and following other simple directions.

The melody of a song such as "This Old Man" makes it easier for your child to learn numbers and the sequential order of events:

This old man, he played one
He played knick-knack with his thumb
With a knick-knack paddy whack, give a dog a bone
This old man came rolling home

This old man, he played two
He played knick-knack with my shoe
With a knick-knack paddy whack, give a dog a bone
This old man came rolling home

This old man, he played three
He played knick-knack on my knee
With a knick-knack paddy whack, give a dog a bone
This old man came rolling home

This old man, he played four
He played knick-knack at my door
With a knick-knack paddy whack, give a dog a bone
This old man came rolling home

This old man, he played five
He played knick-knack jazz and jive

With a knick-knack paddy whack, give a dog a bone
This old man came rolling home

This old man, he played six
He played knick-knack with his sticks
With a knick-knack paddy whack, give a dog a bone
This old man came rolling home

This old man, he played seven
He played knick-knack with his pen
With a knick-knack paddy whack, give a dog a bone
This old man came rolling home

This old man, he played eight
He played knick-knack on my gate
With a knick-knack paddy whack, give a dog a bone
This old man came rolling home

This old man, he played nine
He played knick-knack rise and shine
With a knick-knack paddy whack, give a dog a bone
This old man came rolling home

This old man, he played ten
He played knick-knack in my den
With a knick-knack paddy whack, give a dog a bone
This old man came rolling home

This old man, he played eleven
He played knick-knack up in heaven
With a knick-knack paddy whack, give a dog a bone
This old man came rolling home

This old man, he played twelve
He played knick-knack dig and delve
With a knick-knack paddy whack, give a dog a bone
This old man came rolling home

Four to Five Years: Books

These suggested books have text and story content that are too complex to be interesting to most younger children, and their themes and story events pose and answer increasingly complex questions.

Bob by Tracey Campbell Pearson
Madeline by Ludwig Bemelmans
The Cat in the Hat by Dr. Seuss
One Fish Two Fish Red Fish Blue Fish by Dr. Seuss
The Rose in My Garden by Arnold Lobel
While Mama Had a Quick Little Chat by Amy Reichert

Five to Six Years

As your child begins to read, nursery rhymes can build his vocabulary by introducing him to new words and expressions:

These are Grandma's spectacles
This is Grandma's hat
This is the way she folds her hands
And lays them in her lap

Mary had a little lamb, little lamb, little lamb
Mary had a little lamb, its fleece was white as snow
Everywhere that Mary went, Mary went, Mary went
Everywhere that Mary went, the lamb was sure to go

Your child will be able to use her imagination and play with nursery rhymes now. Practice saying a favorite rhyme the way it was written and then ask your child to help make up an original ending: " 'Jack and Jill went up the hill to fetch a pail of water.' Let's change the ending. 'Jack stubbed his toe and said, "Oh no," and Jill said, "What's the matter?" ' "

Five to Six Years: Books
These recommended books take your child to increasingly imaginative places or show the child's own world from a different perspective.

Agent A to Agent Z by Andy Rash
Good Night, Good Knight by Shelley Moore Thomas
Falling Up by Shel Silverstein
Your Favorite Seuss: A Baker's Dozen by the One and Only Dr. Seuss by Dr. Seuss

NINE

The Skill-Building Value of Play

When you watch a mother cat interact with her growing kittens or a mother dog supervising her puppies, you can see glimpses of the little ones' future in how they play together. A mother cat gently pounces on her babies and lets them go. Her kittens bat at their mother's waving paws and crouch down, stalk, and then spring to attack their mother's flicking tail. A mother dog herds her pups together and encourages them to leap all over her and gently tackle, bite, and nip her and each other and challenge each other for dominance. In the wild the adult cats that kittens become will need to have mastered the skill of stalking. They're also going to need muscle strength and practiced dexterity to pounce on, grab, and hold their prey. Dogs are naturally social animals. In their natural habitat they form packs to hunt and travel in groups. The pups' mother makes sure her babies' roughhousing prepares them for the group activities of an adult dog's life. The animal mothers' interactions with their little ones teach their offspring the skills they'll need in the near future. Cats and dogs don't have classrooms. They don't need them. Like most mammals, our pets understand the value of play.

All children play, too, regardless of the culture they come from or where in the world they live. By playing—alone, with other children, or supervised by their parents—kids learn how to make the fullest and most complete use of the world they live in. Play isn't just a shared experience around the globe; it's a universal need in all children everywhere. Every child needs the time and the opportunity to play creatively and imaginatively each day. For a child with an auditory processing disorder, play becomes a way to express herself freely and spontaneously. It also offers parents a low-pressure and fun way into the child's world that doesn't bring judgment or "shoulds" that a child might find intimidating or frustrating.

PLAYING RULES

The benefits of giving children the gift of creative, age-specific play are almost unlimited. There isn't a single aspect of a child's development that doesn't benefit from creative play. Playing contributes tremendously to a child's physical, emotional, social, and cognitive well-being.

Physical Play
- Athletic games build speed and strength and agility.
- Games involving physical accuracy help a child's motor skills and hand-eye coordination to develop on schedule.
- Hands-on games and play challenge all of a child's senses— sight, sound, smell, taste, and touch—to work together in different combinations.

Emotional Play

- The sense of self-discovery and the feeling of developing expertise and ability that come with playing help a child build and maintain confidence.
- Learning through play accustoms children to the idea that education can be fun. This lesson comes in handy later in life in educational situations where learning becomes difficult.
- Play can teach kids to think their way out of emotionally difficult circumstances.
- Children can deal with stress through play.
- Playing trains children for the rewards of success and accustoms them to the limits of failure.

Social Play

- Playing gives children a chance to exercise and develop their social skills.
- Participation in group dynamics gives children a sense of belonging and fosters empathy.
- Playing with other kids of the same age exposes children to a variety of levels of social abilities and experiences they can model or measure their own against.

Cognitive Play

- Children who use play creatively become good problem solvers.
- Play introduces children to core cognitive concepts such as spatial relationships, cause and effect, the sequences of events, and the passage of time.
- Creative play links thinking with movement and with physically manipulating objects. The phrase "learning how to handle things" has its literal roots in children's early thinking/doing/manipulating experiences while playing.

- Playing draws children to the wealth of details around them, encourages them to make connections between ideas, and spurs them to seek out new things.
- A child's attention span and ability to focus can be improved enormously through games and play activities.

Unfortunately, many parents no longer see the value of play. Recent studies reveal that the amount of time American parents themselves spend playing with their children has dropped to less than forty minutes a week. Compare that to the average forty hours or more that our children are reportedly spending watching television, surfing the Internet, and playing video games. Spending time playing with your child—coming down to meet her at her own eye level and engaging her verbally and physically in an activity you do together—can mean the difference between physical adequacy and athletic prowess, between emotional stability and genuine spirit, between fitting in socially and thriving in a variety of social situations, and between good grades and great grades down the line.

TURNING BACK THE CLOCK

If there's one thing that the twentieth century taught us, it's that technical advances and shortcuts can have a downside. Positive play experiences require that children be allowed to lend as many aspects of their elastic minds as possible to the game or activity at hand. But many modern toys are so specifically engineered and animated that they give a child narrow choices, move the child's imagination into the background, and deny him the pleasure and focusing necessity of personally directing the way that he plays. Toys that move, talk, jump, and flip at the touch of a button make your child a spectator, not a creator. Branded media toys (this includes action figures and toys with the names of TV characters on them) come equipped with a "script" of expectations and story ideas already attached to them. What your child has seen them do on TV dictates how he will play with them. On a purely creative and educational level, it does more good for your child to reenact or imitate what he's seen at the movies or on TV using something unrelated to the exact likeness of the characters he recalls. Pretending a stuffed bear is Dora the Explorer or a sock puppet is Luke Skywalker exercises your child's imagination more than going through the motions with an exact toy likeness.

Human beings are hunter-gatherers in every way. Our minds and curiosities are designed to be stimulated by physical wandering and a varied diet of experience. But safety issues increasingly put our children in controlled environments where beneficially unsupervised play isn't possible. At the same time, accelerated learning programs and the never-ending quest to be prepared for standardized testing have even kindergartners groaning under the weight of extra study and homework. These things have reduced the amount of time children are able to spend playing in school and in some cases even have eliminated or greatly shortened recess time. In a well-intentioned rush to give children every advantage, we have unwittingly narrowed their play options. I'm not asking you to turn your back on any possible school advantage, throw away your television, and let your kids roam the streets. I believe that it's up to parents to set and maintain a balance between creative playtime and the rest of the events in a child's life. As a child grows from infancy to adolescence, exercising that pleasure and privilege brings moms, dads, and kids closer together.

STAGES OF PLAY

Research increasingly details how the progression in complexity in a child's play ritual parallels her mental, physical, and social development. In fact, play activities help to initiate, form, and shape

> *Blake has loved animals since he was a toddler. As he's grown older, they've increasingly become his area of expertise. For years, Blake has enjoyed time spent alone setting up his toy animals on and in the sandbox or the bathtub and creating imaginative scenarios using them. He gets almost as much mileage out of playing with toy knights and castles, mini skateboarding props, and Legos. He enjoys the company of his siblings during his creative and imitative play, and often directs the scenarios with the confidence of someone who's explored and defined his own imaginary story world through private, quiet, and comfortable play.*
>
> —ROSIE

how human beings grow and mature. Just as scaffolding assembled level by level at a building site provides a platform from which to finish each floor of a building, play behavior acts as a stage from which each of us tries out ways to think, communicate, and do things. Throughout a child's development, parents can assist their child in her personal construction job, and help her broaden her experiences and refine and improve her physical, social, and cognitive abilities. The following general guide provides a good starting point for parents and caregivers who want to help their children grow through play.

Infants

Holding, gently rocking, and singing are interactive play activities for infants up to three months. At this early age your child can only see between seven and nine inches in front of him and will play alone and explore those immediate surroundings by waving his limbs and grasping with his fingers and toes. Engage your baby with musical mobiles, wind chimes, or toy mirrors over his crib to stimulate his evolving senses. By three months a baby is usually engaging in rudimentary vocal play. You can join in this activity by responding to his coos and noises. From three to six months your baby will be more awake and active and ready for more play, and between six and nine months, as the difference between sleep and awake time becomes clearly defined, play can be more structured. Look at picture books together and talk to your baby about what the two of you see.

Toddlers

Beginning at nine months, babies show a dramatic increase in what they're able to understand and in their attention span. To help your child begin more challenging play, engage in a game of "show me" and encourage her to point with you. By nine months children also become increasingly interested in colors, sizes, shapes, and sounds—matching, ordering, and comparing them.

From twelve to eighteen months, name objects as you give them to your child and help him group them according to size, color, form, and texture. Talk about the difference between big and small or hot and cold; categorize objects according to what belongs in a group and what does not fit; play peekaboo and other games and activities that encourage comparing and contrasting objects. At this age, human beings are solely focused on their own simple needs. That shouldn't stop you from reading to your child and beginning to model play for him by changing your voice as you read different characters in a story.

Young Preschool: Eighteen to Thirty-Six Months

Preschoolers are fascinated by the material details and qualities of their world. They need play to help discover what "smooth," "scratchy," "bumpy," "brittle," "soft," "elastic," and "fluffy" feel like. These textures will become one of the cornerstones of a foundation of rich and expressive vocabulary. Encourage your child to smell flowers, listen to birds, chase butterflies, and taste freshly picked fruit; offer her words to describe these things. Give her the chance to play with clay, sand, and mud, and play with water together—float toys in a tub, watch ice cubes melt, name all the places you see water (puddle, dog's dish, glass, laundry, tub). Let your child develop a feel for volume and proportion by filling cups, pans, and cans with water or sand and then dumping them out. Preschoolers also become interested in playing with things that will help them understand spatial concepts, including blocks and large-piece puzzles.

This stage is all about relationships and strengthening the bond between you and your child. Your child is ready to play house, so encourage her to come with you around the house and imitate the chores that you do. Give her small tasks and praise her generously and enthusiastically for her efforts. Then reverse roles so that you pretend to be the child and let your child become the parent.

Older Preschool: Three to Five Years

At this stage your child crosses over a threshold into a new realm of the imagination. He is living in a glorious state of consciousness where myth and reality are woven together. His days will now be filled with hours of fantasies, fairy tales, and mysteries. Children this age take their games very seriously and play with a great deal of concentration. They do not have the words to express powerful feelings directly, so they play their way through the issues and increasingly complicated experiences they face. Imaginative play requires props to replace original objects. Your child is hungering for imaginative situations, so be sure to give him the opportunity for creative role-play.

Primary Grades (First, Second, and Third Grades)

Primary school children are learning what makes them unique, and play at this age becomes competitive as children want to demonstrate their unique and defining skills and abilities. Children will make up rules, deliberate, negotiate, and settle upon situations that require some players to change what they're doing in order to keep playing together. This ability to achieve harmony is the foundation of truly social behavior. Grade-schoolers like inventing their own number games and languages and creating secret codes and messages. This kind of play demonstrates a growing understanding of numbers and word meanings.

LISTENING PLAY

All of the component skills of listening that we've explored so far can be addressed and honed through play. Children with APD particularly benefit from listening, language, and speaking games. The physical application of words, their emotional content, and the thought concepts and ideas behind them can all be focused and deepened through play.

Children take ownership of new information and link it to old information through play. Active play fosters personal meaning. When your child makes an event or a fact personally relevant by putting her own spin on it through play, her neural connections increase, and situations, ideas, and skills are ushered into her long-term memory. Think of words and facts as rough clay bowls to a young child. Play shapes these initially crudely defined vessels, smoothes them into specific meanings, bakes them into long-lasting form, glazes them with additional meanings, and, by linking them to other words, facts, and ideas, installs them in a child's long-term memory, where they can be retrieved for multiple uses in multiple ways. Whether a child is struggling with an

A PRIVATE CONVERSATION

When four-year-old Robby comes home from pre-K, his mom gives him a kiss before she heads into the kitchen to warm up a bottle for Robby's new baby brother, Jack. Alone in his room, Robby takes his current favorite toy, a brightly colored earthmover, out of his toy box, and words begin to spill from him like sparkling water from a pitcher. Alternately whispering, giggling, singing, and speaking in a normal voice, Robby talks to himself, the toy, and a combination of characters he's made up and people he knows, such as the school friends he saw in person today and will see again tomorrow. As she sits down to feed her infant son before seeing to her four-year-old's supper, Robby's mom smiles proudly as she hears the private explosion of creativity her little boy is making all on his own.

Robby is engaging in a solo play activity called *private speech.* As they grow older, many children spontaneously begin to talk to themselves during play. Developing children talk out loud to help them figure out what they are going to do and how they are going to do it. They use private speech to practice guiding themselves through challenging situations and to help manage their emotions and impressions of the world inside and outside their heads. Private speech play enables children to face their fears and resolve confusing social, emotional, and reasoning issues. When your child engages in private speech, he is occupying a very important and healthy area of his imagination. The last thing he needs is to be interrupted or questioned as though he were sleepwalking or talking out of turn. When your child loses himself in private speech, let him process his experiences and feelings on his own. Encourage your child to be verbally active in play now, and he's more likely to be able to talk through things and communicate feelings and imaginings later.

APD or not, playing with words and language and using speaking and listening skills in games is the single best way for a child to cultivate her ability to use words and listen.

Young children learn to listen by observing, imitating, and then adapting the examples presented by the world around them. Their natural ability to imitate and repeat what they hear comes so easily that sometimes it might seem like they understand the meaning behind all the words they use. Far from it. In the first three years of life children are not prepared to fully absorb and interpret explanations or descriptions that are beyond their very immediate sense of time, space, and context. By playing and speaking with your child, you help her to attach meanings to the objects she sees and the ideas she uses at play.

LISTENING GAMES AND APD

As we've already discussed, learning is an auditory event that depends strongly on a student's capacity to listen well. That capacity needs to be at its peak when a child enters kindergarten, not just in the process of forming. Cultivating the ability to listen to instructions and follow directions takes years of practice, but there are lots of fun and effective games and exercises to help your children play with words and sounds and learn how to listen.

Listening games are especially helpful for children with an auditory processing disorder. These simple activities do not cost

THE INDIRECT CONNECTION

An adult speaks to a one- to three-year-old child in two ways:

- Direct language asks the child testing questions and issues commands.
- Indirect language requires no specific response and offers your child a more nuanced and adaptable speaking example to model his own language after.

Modeling indirect language for your child is much better than direct language for his developing listening skills and ongoing ability to learn, integrate, and store the information and word meanings he hears.

Talk about the action your child performs, what an object is, and a detail that defines it, or narrate what you are doing, all using simple, four- or five-word sentences:

"You're playing with a truck."
"You're making it go."
"There's a tree. It's a big tree."
"I'm cooking. Mmm, smells good."

Incorporate expansion and extension—when your child says something, confirm what she or he has said and add a little more.

Your child: "Plane."
You: "Yes, it's a red plane."
Your child: "Want apple."
You: "Do you want a piece of apple?"

> Expand your child's short phrase into a brief, grammatically correct sentence:
>
> Your child: "Truck."
> You: "You have a big blue truck."

anything and can be done virtually anywhere—at home, in the car, at the grocery store, or waiting in a doctor's office.

What do you hear? Ask your child to close her eyes and listen carefully. What kinds of sounds does she hear?

Name that sound. Ask your child to close her eyes. Use ordinary objects that make different sounds, such as a toy cow that moos and a bird toy that chirps, and ask her to identify what she hears. Then close your eyes and let your child choose sounds for you to identify, too.

Follow the musical leader. Sing or hum part of a song that your child knows, and ask her to repeat it.

Bedtime review. As your child gets ready for bed, ask her to recount what she did that day. Can your child recall the events sequentially?

These games can be used individually to target an area that is weak in a child's listening skill set or as a set to strengthen the entire developmental range of a child's auditory skills.

Games for Children Two to Four Years Old

These games are generally appropriate for two-, three-, and four-year-olds (though certain eighteen-month-olds will be able to play some of them).

Show Me

This game helps a child listen and follow directions.

At an early age you must say and do each action. Later you and your child can say and do it together.

"Show me how you touch your nose."
"Show me up on tippy toes."
"Show me how you bend your knees."
"Show me how you buzz like bees."

Make them up as you go; they don't have to rhyme. "Show me how you put your hands on hips."

After you play a few times and your child gets a little older, you may not have to demonstrate; you can just give the verbal direction.

A variation is to make up silly directions: "Show me how you put your ear to the floor." Remember, kids like being silly.

Going on a Sound Walk

Take a walk outside and listen for the sounds around you. Here are a few ideas:

People talking
Horns beeping
Wind blowing
Your footsteps (in leaves, in snow)
Dogs barking
Sirens

Talk about the sounds and imitate them just for fun.
This same activity can be played in the house.

Listening Farmyard Fun

Use toy farm animal figures and say the sounds each one makes. Now ask your child to close his eyes. Make an animal sound. When your child opens his eyes, ask him to show you which animal he heard.

Try three other animals. Then turn the game around and have your child make the sound and you pick the animal.

Listening Identification

Pick a word such as "cat" that has a distinctive sound associated with it and tell your child to say "meow, meow" every time she hears the word "cat": "Dog, cat, man, house, flow, cat, blue, yellow, cat . . ."

Change the word to "car." Ask your child to say "beep-beep" when she hears "car," and say a list of words with "car" sprinkled in.

Fill in the Blank

Sing a song to your child such as "Row, Row, Row Your Boat." Do it a few times softly, and then on the third go-round, sing the word "boat" louder: "Row, row, row your **boat** . . ."

Next time you sing it pause before the word "boat" to invite your child to fill in the word. Once your child understands the game, try the second line, and continue until you have completed the song.

Whispering Wisps

Say a phrase to your child in a normal voice: "It is morning." Now say the same phrase in a whisper. Ask your child if he can say it in a whisper.

Now ask questions in a whisper: "What's your name?" See if

your child can answer you in a whisper. Pretty soon you will be having a whole conversation in a whisper.

Can I Have . . .

In this game the child has to listen and get you the item you ask for. Children love to listen and find.

> "Can I please have . . . the ball?"
> . . . the shoe?"
> . . . the bear?"

Remember to say thank you when your child gives you the item you requested.

Telephone Talk

Make up a conversation using two toy telephones or a reasonable imitation.

> You: "Hello?"
> Your child: "Hello."
> You: "What are you doing today?"
> Your child: "Playing."

Ask who, what, why, where, and when questions that require thinking up an answer, not just saying yes or no.

Variations: See if your child can ask you a question. Pretend to call other people. Make believe you are other people.

Listening for Patterns

Have several children line up and make a "train." Tell them you are going to blow a whistle and that one short whistle means "stop" and two short whistles means "go slow"; demonstrate each. As they chug around the room together, blow the whistle to make them stop and slow down. Once they can handle two instructions, add a third: three whistles means "back up" and one long whistle means "stop and turn around."

Do What I Say

Have your child collect two or three stuffed animals. Tell him to carry out each instruction you give with the animal named. Call on each animal. "Mr. Bear?" (Your child gets the bear.) "Go to sleep." (Your child puts the bear down as if sleeping.) "Miss Duck, jump up and down." Now switch roles.

Guess What I Am

One child chooses a person, place, or thing. To make this game easier, you can have five pictures out for the child to choose from. The other children, or a parent, asks questions:

"Are you red?"
"Do you float?"
"Do you have a string?"

The first child answers yes or no depending on what she is thinking of. The first one to guess correctly wins.

Musical Chairs

Put out as many chairs as there are children. Play music. The children circle the chairs while the music is playing. When the music stops they must find a chair and sit until the music begins again. With young children there should always be enough chairs. For older children you can have one chair less than the number of children, and the child without a seat is out.

A variation: Play lively music. Pass a beanbag around a circle of children. When the music stops, the child holding the beanbag is out.

Duck, Duck, Goose

All the players sit in a circle. One person is chosen as "it." She walks on the outside of the circle, tapping each child gently on the head, saying "duck . . . duck . . . duck . . ." When she says "goose" the child she has tapped gets up and chases her. She must try to get to the empty spot and sit down before being tagged. If she makes it, the goose becomes "it."

Simon Says

One person is chosen as "Simon." He stands in front of the group and tells the group what to do: "Simon says touch your toes. Simon says touch your nose."

The players must follow the directions only if "Simon" says "Simon says" before he gives the direction. If Simon does not say "Simon says" first—for example, just "Touch your knees"—and a player does it anyway, she is out.

My Grandma Has a Grocery Store

This is a great game for auditory sequential memory. The first player starts with the letter "A" and finishes the following sentence with a word that begins with that letter: "My grandma owns a grocery store and she sells . . . apples."

As you go back and forth or from child to child, each player repeats the previous answers and adds an item that begins with the next letter in the alphabet: "My grandma owns a grocery store and she sells apples and bananas." "My grandma owns a grocery store and she sells apples and bananas and carrots."

If someone misses, you can give clues to keep the game going, or that person can be out.

Role-Playing

Pretend together, picking as many activities as you can: "What kinds of things can we pretend?" One person guesses what the other is doing. Some examples:

> Feeding a doll
> Combing your hair
> Driving a car
> Washing your face
> Climbing a ladder
> Drawing a picture

Yes, No, Maybe So

Ask your child to answer "yes," "no," or "maybe so" to your questions.

> "Is the sky blue?"
> "Do you wear ice skates to bed?"
> "Do pants talk?"
> "Do boats cry?"
> "Do cats bark?"
> "Are bananas purple?"

> The sillier the question, the better!

Fun for Five-Year-Olds

These games are appropriate for five-year-olds.

Eating the Alphabet

Pick a letter for the day—say, "A." Tell your child, "Let's name all the things we can eat that start with 'A.' " Make a list together:

applesauce, apples, apricots, artichokes, almonds, avocados . . . The next day, see how many you can remember.

Pick a different letter each day. Or start at the end of the alphabet and go backward!

To Market, to Market

Say, "Let's make a shopping list. I'll remember five things and you remember five things." Write a list together and hide it in your pocket before you go to the grocery store. No peeking until checkout time.

Tick Tock, Tick Tock: Where's the Clock?

Hide a timer or a ticking clock somewhere in the room, then have your child come into the room. She must listen carefully and try to find the timer or clock by following the sound. Give hints if needed: "cold" if far away, "warm" or "warmer" if nearer, "hot" if very close.

TEN

Nurturing Social Skills: The Listening-Speaking-Relating Connection

It's lunchtime during a school field trip to the local planetarium. It was a drizzly morning, but while seven-year-old Jennifer and her classmates were inside looking across the universe, the sun came out and it turned into a beautiful spring day. Sitting at a picnic table next to a statue of Galileo, Jennifer tears into a bag of potato chips her mom put in her lunch. Jennifer's classmate Miriam looks at them enviously from across the table. Jennifer has a hard time reading people's expressions sometimes and it's been a big, noisy day so far. Not really sure what Miriam wants, at first Jennifer shyly ignores her and looks away. Finally Miriam reaches out for Jennifer's chip bag.

"Can I have some?" Miriam asks.

Jennifer looks at her and cocks her head. "You're silly!" she answers.

"No I'm not," Miriam says.

"You are too!" Jennifer replies, laughing. "What you said is silly."

"What is?" Miriam has no idea what she means.

"You want a son?" Jennifer says.

"What?" Miriam's caught by surprise. She just wanted to engage her classmate and have some potato chips, not get made fun of.

"That's silly!" Jennifer laughs at the idea.

"But that's not what I said!" Miriam says.

"It is!" Jennifer squeals.

"No it's not. That's not what I said!"

Jennifer's getting frustrated. She knows what she heard. "It is too!"

"No, I said I want some chips."

Now Jennifer is getting confused. She heard what she heard. "You didn't say that!" she says shrilly.

"Yes I did!"

"No you did not!" Jennifer's yelling now. "You did not!" Jennifer throws the chips down on the table between them, scaring Miriam. Their teacher arrives and separates the two girls. Miriam is crying.

"What happened, Jennifer?" the teacher asks. This is not the first time Jennifer's been in a situation like this. She's trying to make friends, but blowups like this are getting more and more frequent. Just like the last time, Jennifer says nothing. Her feelings are hurt, just like Miriam's, but instead of crying she withdraws.

"Jennifer, what happened?" the teacher asks again. "What did you say to her?"

Her teacher makes a mental note to mention to Jennifer's parents that their daughter is increasingly socially combative with her peers and withdrawn in social situations with adults. These aren't good signs. Her teacher is beginning to suspect that Jennifer needs to be screened for a behavioral problem by a psychologist and that Jennifer's parents have a tough road ahead of them.

SOCIAL LEARNING

We've looked at how children's listening abilities impact their education and at what parents can do to help their kids prepare for that aspect of their listening lives. But structured learning and the passing of knowledge from teacher to student is only one-half of the experience of education. The other, equally important side of that coin is the experience of social interaction, which goes along with academics and parallels school-age development. The line between social interactions and educational interactions is a blurred one. So much of what we expect our children to learn is tested, fine-tuned, and reinforced by their play and conversations with each other before, during, and after school.

It's worth mentioning that we don't send our children to nursery school and pre-K to teach them to read and write. The developmental goal of preschool education is almost entirely social. Yes, your preschool child learns songs and rhymes and games, but more than anything else pre-primary education is designed to expose your child to the social rituals of education—listening to and answering questions, working in groups with peers, taking turns, and learning the boundaries between okay and not-okay behavior. As a child follows nursery school with pre-K and then goes on to kindergarten and first grade, the social importance of going to school grows along with academic responsibilities.

Communication can be a fragile thing, especially for children. As a child grows from infancy to school age, his need to establish and maintain two-way social communication with the people who inhabit the world around him becomes greater and greater. As adults, we take the rituals of conversation for granted. It's easy to forget that each of us has had to learn how to conduct a verbal dialogue with others, just as we learned to tie our shoes, read, or drive. Social communication is in its most basic form an alternation between speaking and listening. We've all experienced the frustration of being interrupted, ignored, or marginalized in a conversation by a person who won't let us get a word in edgewise.

For a child who, like Jennifer in the story above, lacks the listening skill to participate in a social conversation, that frustration—the feeling of being left out, unheard, pushed aside—can be a daily burden. Social skills are based in listening skills. Children with strong social skills can gain more from both classroom and playground activities. They have a distinct advantage in nearly every arena. When a child can't listen, he can't sustain social connections. Whether due to an APD or other developmental condition, children who struggle with listening are almost guaranteed to struggle also with the challenges of interacting with their peers, fitting in, and making friends.

Words, their meanings, and our rituals of language are what connect us to each other. If your child struggles to connect with words, he will have the same difficulty connecting with people. The cornerstone of adequate, age-appropriate social ability is listening. Jennifer has had difficulty listening since she was a toddler, but when she was smaller the social expectations were not very demanding. As children get older they need the grounding and self-defining pleasure, challenge, and variety of both one-on-one and group social exchanges in order to mature, function, and participate in our communication-intensive society. Jennifer is falling behind in a socially driven world that expects her to listen to language and learn the rituals that surround it.

Jennifer has an undiagnosed APD. Instead of meeting the developmental challenge of social interaction, she finds herself getting into more and more trouble as she tries to hold up her end of any conversation. Her obligation to listen is growing, but her ability to do it well isn't. Jennifer's a sensitive girl and a smart one. She needs the same things that all children get out of social interactions, whether in the schoolroom or the schoolyard: attention, the reassuring companionship of other children their age, and the sense of safety that comes from connecting with the adults in their lives. Increasingly, Jennifer gets neither. Worse, when she tries to participate, much of the time the result is bad. The conventional avenue to getting attention doesn't work, so she unconsciously starts pursuing other ways of getting attention, including aggressive behavior and tantrums. Her teachers and caregivers see only the acting-out behavior, not the need for attention that unconsciously motivates it, nor the inability to listen that leads Jennifer to act this way in the first place.

By age six or seven most children need to be able to apply the basic social skills listed below. These skills all have a listening component. Children with APD may have missed the words to go with these skills or are unaware of the cues that trigger these types of responses.

- Taking turns speaking. A child with APD may not recognize the auditory signals for when it is her turn to speak.
- Staying on task and completing assigned activities. A child with APD may be distracted by environmental sounds or may not have heard the complete directions to an assignment in accurate and full enough detail to do it satisfactorily.
- Sharing material. A child with APD often does not understand or know how to use the permission and engagement of the language of sharing: "Can I play with you?" "Can I have a turn?" "I want to play by myself."
- Using another person's name. A child with APD may not have attached the right name to a person, may not have heard the name itself accurately, may not have realized that a specific person's name is relevant information, or may have forgotten the name altogether.
- Waiting for a turn. The APD child may miss the verbal signals for turn taking in games and play.

- Listening actively. A child with APD may have difficulty staying engaged in a conversation or conversation-based activity because the language and information is too complex and confusing or the situation itself is too noisy.

- Following directions. The APD child may have difficulty following through due to struggles with auditory memory or auditory sequential memory. Steps in sequences of directions can be left out, confused with one another, or followed out of order.

- Sharing ideas. Struggling with APD or similar listening issues can rob a child of necessary vocabulary and the ability to distinguish similar-sounding words. That child may have difficulty keeping up in a conversation.

- Participating equally with others. Again, a child with an APD can misread signals and lack the level of language peers use. Such a child will likely withdraw from a group activity or conversation, perform badly, or find some other, potentially inappropriate way to participate.

- Initiating a topic. A child needs to come to a shared experience with the necessary vocabulary and experience to use her words.

- Maintaining a topic. That same vocabulary and confidence enable a child to continue a conversation.

- Asking and answering conversational questions. A child with APD may not understand how to formulate a question. He may struggle with intonation and be unable to comprehend or identify the specific uses and differences between yes/no questions and who, what, where, when, and why questions.

- Recognizing and responding to the feelings of others. A child with APD may not have the words to express appropriate feelings to match the situation or be able to "read" the emotional intonations in what's being said to her.

- Successfully entering a group. A child with APD often is so confused by group conversation or has so much difficulty following what's being said by many different voices that he chooses not to participate.
- Asking for, offering, and giving help. The child struggling with APD may not be aware of when she needs help or the appropriate way to gain another's attention if she does. She may misread the signs and words associated with another child's need for help and may lack the vocabulary to give verbal instructions.

All of these social abilities increasingly come into play on the road to adulthood. What also unites these skills is that they are all based on listening. And listening, as we've already discussed, is an evolving process of skill building all its own. As we've seen, listening—the active application of hearing—begins at birth. Listening skills and social skills are so completely intertwined that as children lay the groundwork for listening, they also start to form the foundation of the social skills that they will use listening for. To understand how to help equip your child with the social skills she will need, and how to help her learn ways to deal with listening-based social problems, it's a good idea to look at how social skills evolve and develop in concert with the ability to listen. If a child's listening skills are slowed by an APD, her social skills undoubtedly will suffer, too.

TEACHING BY EXAMPLE

We recognize the beginnings of individual personality in our children from our first days together. But who our children are and how they relate to us and to the other people around them develop over time. Long before they have teachers in school, our kids are getting a crash course in how the world works, who they are, and how to behave from their first and most important teachers—their parents. Psychologists call it *modeling*—our children base their own behavior on the feedback they get from us in the millions of interactions, big and small, we share throughout the day. Children model their behavior after ours and demonstrate what they're learning as they do it. You are always teaching your child by talking to him, interacting, and playing with him. It's these examples that he uses when trying out social behavior appropriate to each stage of his development. As with all of the developmental descriptions used in this book, the typical responses and building blocks of social skills and listening described below are general. They're based on my clinical experience and on the results of research done by others in the field of child development and speech-language pathology. No child hits all of these stages and crosses each of the growth thresholds on cue. This is meant as a primer to help you better understand your role in your child's social development, not a checklist for how a child should behave at any given age. A working knowledge of how social skills develop will help you to be more attentive to your child's responses and actively encourage his evolving skills.

Birth to One Year

During this first year together with your baby, you'll do all the talking. A newborn is wide open to hearing language—inflection, syllables, component phonemes, volume—yet unable to do much in the way of talking back. But she is listening, and she's letting you know it. Initially your baby's social responses are primarily physical. She will react to physical attention. When picked up and held, your baby will either wriggle or mold her body to yours. But despite not being able to form language yet, she is still keenly attuned to hearing it. Unless there's an auditory problem—either a difficulty hearing or a difficulty processing what is heard—over the course of the first year she will begin to have her half of the "conversation" by being attentive to you when you speak, making sounds, and returning eye contact.

Two to Four Months
The baby will return smiles and laughs and can gaze at people alertly.

Three to Six Months
An infant is able to vocally express both pleasure and displeasure distinctly.

Four to Six Months
A baby shows he is aware of new or different surroundings and will quiet down to the reassuring voice of a parent. The baby will also begin passively enjoying social "play" by smiling when you make noises at him, keeping his attention on you when you talk to him, and noticing when you enter or leave the room. Children with APD can be slow to react or may do so inconsistently.

Four to Seven Months
Through sounds and gestures, your baby demands your attention in the same way she demands food.

Four to Eight Months
At some point during this period, most babies will begin to return the vocalizing you direct at them, babbling, cooing, or making other noises.

Five to Eight Months
Babies begin independently playing with their own vocal abilities and listening to the sounds they produce.

Five to Nine Months
Your baby recognizes and reaches for you and other caregivers.

Six to Eleven Months
He now makes noises for attention. Your baby has noticed that when he cries, he gets picked up or fed and that his voice has power. He's already begun to define and test parental limits physically by throwing things from his high chair, playing with food, and so on. Now he uses his voice and his hearing to explore the nature of his relationship with you by crying out or continuing to do something after being told no.

Seven to Twelve Months
The beginnings of active play. Play peekaboo by using a baby blanket to cover your face momentarily, then uncover it. At this stage, after a few turns your child isn't just watching; she's expecting you to reappear each time—so much so that if you pause and stay hidden, she'll squeal or reach for the blanket.

Eight to Twelve Months
Your child starts to imitate noises, syllables, and even words he hears.

Ten to Twelve Months
Your child shows and offers toys or other objects to her parents.

Eleven to Twelve Months
When you make a sound at your baby, he will make a sound back at you and the two of you can keep the exchange up for several turns. This back-and-forth in which your child recognizes that he is being heard and responded to is the dawning of conversation. This stage can arrive earlier or later, but if this back-and-

forth dynamic never really takes root, it can be a red flag indicating that there may be something wrong in the way your child processes sound.

Age One to Two

Now your child begins to build words out of the sounds she hears and incorporate them into your exchanges. The one- to two-year-old's half of the "conversation" may just be a single word or word-like sound. You need to listen for these early words and use them in the sentences you say and the questions you ask to vertically attach more words and horizontally add meaning. When your baby says, "Ball," for example, you could respond with, "Yes, that is a ball," "Can you roll the ball?" "See how I roll it?" or "It rolls because it's round."

Twelve to Eighteen Months
Baby imitates new words.

Twelve to Nineteen Months
He or she can independently express approximately five to ten words.

Thirteen to Fifteen Months
By this stage your baby can successfully hand you a toy or other object and even manage a give-and-take of the object between you. Inviting you to play in this way sets the stage for initiating social interactions and conversations.

Thirteen to Eighteen Months
The beginnings of your child's sense of humor start to emerge, and your verbal exchanges can be silly and done "just for laughs."

TEACHING SOCIAL SKILLS

1. Concentrate on one skill at a time. When learning skills, most children find it difficult to focus on too many new things at once. Children learn social behavior by modeling what they do after behavior they've seen. If they are old enough to brainstorm ideas with you, discuss the skill and how it might be used. If your child is not mature enough, tell her exactly what to do and to say. For example, if you're working on the skill of asking for help, seek your child's assistance while coloring together: "Chloe, I need a pink crayon. Can you help me find one? . . . Oh, thank you, that's just the one I needed!"

2. Give praise. "You are such a good helper." Or give a thumbs-up and a smile.

3. Remind your child during the day of how she helped you earlier and take opportunities to praise her when she uses a social skill appropriately: "I liked the way you waited your turn in the game before."

4. Use reading. There are many books appropriate to various age groups that deal with social skills. Seeing and hearing characters overcome obstacles and learn how to use skills successfully sets the right example to follow. Browse the shelves at your library and see if there's a book for a social skill that you feel your child could improve.

5. While watching a movie with your child, comment on things the characters do or say that were appropriate or inappropriate to the situation. Ask what your child thinks.

6. Eye contact, facial expression, body posture, proximity, movement clarity, and tone of voice are all important parts of social skills. Make sure to incorporate the necessary physical cues for a social skill into your teaching time.

7. The best solution for building your child's social skills is to role-play with her. Pretend you are a similar-age peer and set up the situation that needs work. Role-playing together helps your child develop comfort and ability with her new knowledge and skills in a safe environment.

8. Once you have learned the skill together, move on to the next one, but be sure to practice what you've already mastered.

Fifteen to Twenty-three Months

She displays affection for you and for other people by hugging and kissing and throwing kisses.

Eighteen to Twenty-four Months

By now your child's expressive vocabulary has expanded to approximately twenty words.

Nineteen to Twenty-four Months

Your baby can play alongside other infants his age. As a child approaches age two he demonstrates a wide range of emotions on his face, including happiness, sadness, fear, frustration, and concern.

Age Two to Three

The "terrible twos" are actually a time of incredible growth in your child's social life. During this year he expresses his natural need for control and desire for independence by going where he wants, grabbing things, and saying no to get attention. He may be exhausting to keep up with and clean up after, and all those nos and struggling can feel pretty monotonous and negative, but it's a social and developmental period a child has to go through to find the power of language and how to function in social interactions.

Twenty-three to Thirty-two Months
During these months your child can use approximately fifty words independently in verbal exchanges.

Twenty-four to Thirty Months
Your toddler begins to empathize and identify feelings in other people that she has herself. She will attempt to comfort other people when she senses they are upset. Hugging Mom's leg or another toddler her age who is crying is meant to make both of you feel better. An inability to empathize, or consistent confusion about and disinterest in the emotional responses of others, can indicate that a child isn't taking in everything she is hearing.

Twenty-four to Thirty Months
Your child begins to use social language by commenting and responding to greetings and requests. He uses specific words to gain attention, rather than just saying things loudly or over and over.

Twenty-four to Thirty-one Months
He has become better at linking words with melodies and rhythm in songs and rhymes. He can recognize a familiar song by the words and tune, or just the tune.

Twenty-five to Thirty Months
Your toddler can appear shy with strangers and in new situations.

Twenty-five to Thirty Months
Increasingly a child at this age demonstrates enjoyment of his relationships with others. He looks forward to seeing specific people, getting their attention, and making them laugh.

Twenty-five to Thirty-six Months
Your toddler has assembled the social skills necessary to interactively play with one other child.

Thirty to Thirty-six Months
Your child is able to play interactively with one other child.

Thirty to Thirty-six Months
Your child talks to you when you read to her.

Thirty-two to Thirty-six Months
Brief conversations begin. The child's expressive vocabulary is approaching two hundred words or more.

Thirty-four to Thirty-Six Months
Building on the prior years of studying inflection, your child can now answer yes/no questions and who, what, where, when, and why questions with increasing confidence and ease. He's also using words to describe his emotions and the emotions of others.

Age Three to Four

At about three years of age, your child learns a simple lesson about time and the art of conversation, one that children with an auditory processing disorder often miss. If you have been modeling speech frequently and leaving time for even your infant child to answer, by now your child will pick up on a central component of turn taking. He's learned in the past three years of watching, listening, and playing with you that a pause greater than one second means that he is not likely to get a response from whomever he is speaking with. By the same token, a short pause of less than one second lets him know that the topic is still being talked about. Armed with this ability to define his part in a conversation, his experience with reading people's voices and expressions, and his increased vocabulary, urging your child to "use his words" instead of acting out starts to mean something.

Thirty-six to Forty-two Months
By this point children can be using between three hundred and one thousand words of expressive vocabulary.

Thirty-six to Forty-eight Months
A child begins to use verbal reprimands such as "no" or "give it" instead of pushing, grabbing, or being physically aggressive.

Thirty-seven to Forty Months
Your child is beginning to play interactively with a small group of her peers.

Thirty-seven to Forty-eight Months
In one-on-one or group play, your child becomes able to ask permission to use a toy that another child has. She also begins to follow rules based on imitating actions of those closest to her. If she is encouraged consistently, for instance, her requests during this period can evolve from "I want" and "gimme" to "may I" or "can I."

Forty-two to Forty-eight Months
The balance necessary for conversation becomes more defined for a child this age. By now he is learning the rudiments of turn tak-

SOCIAL BREAKDOWNS

Your child may have different auditory skills than her peers. She may not be able to keep up with the conversation. She may have extra difficulty listening to and comprehending what another person has said to her, and she may not be able to respond appropriately. An APD or other listening problem can be the root cause of any of the following:

- Inability to successfully enter a group. Some children haven't yet learned the words that admit them to group activities: "What are you playing?" "My name's Micah," "I like dinosaurs, too," "Can I play?"
- Inability to successfully follow directions. When another child gives the directions for play, a child who can't process the words will mess up repeatedly and leave frustrated.
- Inability to stay on or maintain a topic of conversation or topic of play. Children with an APD may rush to change the topic to what they want to talk about because it is easier for them to talk than to listen.
- Unfamiliarity with the rules of play. Turn taking and the reciprocal cycle of play need to be learned and mastered.
- Lack of awareness of others' feelings. Children cut off from listening are sometimes also cut off from the emotional effects of the things they do.

ing—the application of words, pausing, listening, and following through—that are necessary for two-way talk.

Forty-three to Forty-eight Months

Your child is beginning to answer more complex questions having two parts and involving speculation and other things not immediately at hand: "Would you like to go to the zoo? What kinds of animals do you think we'll see there?"

Age Four to Five

Over the past twelve months your child has learned how to use pauses in conversation as a cue for initiating his turn to speak. He has also been initiated into the difficulties of simultaneous talking and interruption and will now give up a turn to speak in order to keep an interesting or emotionally engaging conversation going. A child with this degree of social skills—able to take turns, talk, and listen—is ready for kindergarten.

Forty-eight to Sixty Months
Your child can take turns speaking and listening in larger groups of children. Asking permission to use toys or other objects that belong to or are held by others becomes more automatic. She can repeat or recite songs, rhymes, or dances for others, without having to do them along with you. She can also contribute to adult conversations when invited.

Fifty-four to Sixty Months
By this point your child's social skills are put to good use as he gravitates toward his own peers much more than toward you and other adults. He can accomplish tasks together with his peers and work in small groups for ten to twenty-five minutes at a time. Failure and disappointment have clear definitions and verbal reactions associated with them, and who, what, where, when, and why questions are answered with even more specificity. Your child's ability to name and categorize items and objects deepens, and he can repeat back multiple-word sentences.

THE ART OF CONVERSATION

At its core, social communication is built on good conversation. I don't mean lively or informative conversation, though that is a worthwhile goal in itself. Good conversation, the kind that forms the basis of strong social skills, is simply a clear alternating between talking and listening. We have all enjoyed the pleasure of sharing in conversations that hold our attention and engage us intellectually. We all also know the feeling of being trapped in conversations that are meaninglessly repetitive or confusing, or in which we don't seem to be able to make ourselves clear or understood.

Current studies indicate that adults only attend to about 50 percent of what's said in most conversations. Also, most of us can attend to what's being said in any given conversation for only about twenty minutes at a time, and that figure dips far lower when we're tired or under a lot of stress. Taking turns in conversation and keeping a specific conversational topic going are skills that grow as children do. On average, a developing child's ability to maintain a conversational topic begins to take shape in the first two or three years of life, so somewhere between age two and three most kids can manage two turns in a conversation on most topics:

> You: "Do you want to come to the market?"
> Your child: "Yes please."
> You: "Is there anything special you want to get while we're there?"
> Your child: "Cereal! And ice cream!"

Of course, if the topic is of particular interest to him, your child will likely go many more turns, but at that age, two times is fairly average. By age five the number of turns grows to about five, including repeating all or part of what has been said to him, or asking questions of his own to clarify what he's heard. The average adult should be able to sustain a conversation for about eleven turns. And yet increasingly in our shorthand-obsessed society, where technology inclines us to keep communications brief and we are bombarded with repetitive and meaningless verbiage from advertising, many grown men and women can only manage a conversational exchange of two to three turns—about average for a four-year-old! If we want our children to get the most out of their education and out of the simple and universal pleasure of interacting with the people around them, we need to set them the best conversational example we can.

The basic rules for teaching good conversation are the same whether we are participating in conversation with a child or an adult.

Pay Attention

Respect your child's attempts to connect with you, whether it's a newborn's gaze and happy burbling, an older infant handing you a cup or toy, a two-year-old enjoying story time by talking about the story you read to her, a four-year-old describing a dream, or a five-year-old sharing a secret.

Really Listen

Even with newborns, leave pauses to gauge your child's reaction to what you do and say. Making spaces for a reaction or contribution is one of the only ways to make possible reciprocity—the return volley of language you initiate or pick up.

Stay on Topic

Depending on how old your child is, she can keep up her side of a conversation only so long. Don't make it even harder for her by trying to discuss two things at once, skipping back to prior topics without any setup or warning, or piling too many instructions into one sentence. As much as possible, let her lead the conversation and follow the topic where she wishes to take it.

Use *Your* Words, Mom and Dad!

As you narrate what you're doing together with an infant, describe sights and experiences with your toddler, or talk through more complex activities with an older child, use words that clearly describe how the objects, processes, and results you share look, feel, taste, and smell. Remember that you are teaching when you're talking, whether you intend to or not. Using vague or needlessly complex language is going to leave your child looking for words rather than give him what he needs.

Use Your Body

Be conscious of keeping eye contact, making reassuring gestures and facial expressions, and using your body posture and proximity to make yourself accessible to your child at her level. She'll read these cues with increasing skill if she has a consistent and expressive example to follow.

Words Have Feelings

Help your child understand his own feelings and emotions and appreciate how important other people's feelings are by using words that describe emotions and their function. The emotional world of a child is a powerful thing. The joys and fears of childhood can be overwhelming if your child can't describe what he is feeling or talk about how the people around him feel. Remember that a young child tends to measure emotional experiences in

> *Working on empathy is a big thing. Empathy needs to be learned and it needs to be witnessed—it needs to be felt and it needs to be implemented. When your kids are empathetic on their own, when they share and are willing to share and help if somebody is hurt, make a big deal out of it. Let them know how other people's displays of emotion make you feel. You have to really point out to kids the things that other people do that you want to see repeated and reflected and imitated in your kids' behavior.*
>
> —ROSIE

terms of cause and effect, so use this approach to his feelings and the feelings of others as you help him learn how to use conversation to navigate his own emotional world and to empathize with others. "You seem sad. Are you sad because it is time to stop playing?" "I think the fish in the story was happy because he found his mother. What do you think?"

Empathy Needs Help

Empathy puts us in another person's shoes. Empathy is not feeling sorry for someone; it is simply understanding the feelings the other person has. Children learn empathy by modeling their behavior on that of their parents and other adults. They need the example, and they also need the words and concepts that help them identify, describe, and understand their feelings. A child experiences empathy as cause and effect—how her actions and words affect a friend or a sibling. True empathy can be hard for anyone. In order to function and experience emotional connection with other people, we all have to escape the infantile stage of thinking that the world revolves around us. A child with an APD can become cut off from the emotional meaning of words and the feeling that comes with the way they are said. It's especially important to teach empathy to children whose social skills have been affected by an inability to listen well. Reward acts of kindness when your child demonstrates them. Explain the reason for another person's tears, laughter, or other emotional state. Give children the room and the time to describe what the cause and effect of their emotional state is, and encourage them to speculate about others.

ELEVEN

The Magic of Reading:
Using Books to Build Listening
and Critical-Thinking Skills

Reading is a magical experience that opens up a whole new world of wonder. Stories can transport us to places that exist far outside the boundaries of ordinary reality and carry us through enchanted landscapes where anything is possible. Through the words, images, and ideas contained in a book, children can fly through the starry skies, talk to wild animals, build an igloo, ride on a whale, and leap over skyscrapers. Books allow us to travel back through time, to when dinosaurs walked the earth, or soar into the future, journeying through the farthest reaches of space.

But reading provides children with so much more than a window into the imagination. Books expand their perspective of the world and allow them to experience new concepts they would not otherwise encounter. Hearing stories read aloud is also one of the most powerful ways for children to develop strong listening and language skills.

Reading is an acquired skill that your child must gradually

learn how to do and an art that has to be cultivated and practiced over time. Though it will take your child years to learn how to read a book himself, he is ready to hear you read to him from almost the beginning of his life. As he grows and the two of you continue to share the experience of reading together, the bond you share will grow, too. Being read to from an early age conditions your child's brain to associate the act of reading with pleasure. And children who enjoy books have a greater desire to learn how to read on their own.

The rewards of reading are so rich that I ask all the parents I work with to establish their own reading ritual with their child. In this chapter, I'll share some of the best tips I've found for reading a story to a child, and help you choose books that will educate, entertain, and inspire your son or daughter for many years to come.

It is really never too early to begin reading to your child. Babies respond to the sound of your voice from the moment they are born. As we've seen, infants need to hear language spoken long before they develop the capacity to understand words. In time, toddlers start to associate words with pictures in books and make a meaningful connection between what they hear and what they see on the page. This is a giant and very necessary step in the growth and development of your child's listening skills.

The reading ritual and special time that you share does not have to stop once children learn how to read on their own. It is a wonderful idea to continue sharing stories with fourth, fifth, and sixth graders, and even beyond. Adults even enjoy being read to once in a while, too.

As your child learns to read on his own, read one chapter together each week or take turns reading from a book that he otherwise would not be ready to understand on his own. There are many classic works that will build your child's vocabulary and explore the timeless challenges he is experiencing.

Reading is one of the most joyful bonding experiences that parents can share with their children. It offers an opportunity to achieve a unique harmony. Through sharing books we can stop, relax for a few moments, and just be with our children. Stories bring us together and help us to understand one another on a level that is deeply nurturing and comforting. All that is required is a willingness to listen.

And yet it's estimated that only 20 percent of parents read to their children on a daily basis. We have become so busy trying to manage all the activities in our lives that we are losing opportunities to connect with our children in one of the most meaningful and beneficial ways available to us.

WHY READING IS SO IMPORTANT FOR APD

The time you spend reading can be a dynamic listening and language lesson that will enable your child to build specific skills. There are very simple reading exercises that you can do to strengthen a child's auditory memory, auditory sequencing, and auditory cohesion. These are some of the prerequisite skills that all children need in order to read on their own. For a child with an auditory processing disorder, reading aloud is a way of hearing and learning vocabulary with built-in visual support.

Auditory Memory

Auditory memory is the ability we need to retain and recall information that we hear through listening. There are many books that can help your child develop this skill. Here are suggestions for strengthening auditory memory using *The Gingerbread Man* by Catherine McCafferty.

- Begin by reading the book for pleasure without asking any questions. Take the time to look at the book's colorful pictures with your child as you focus on the story.
- The second time you read the book, say something like this: "There are a lot of characters who are hungry and who want to eat the gingerbread man. Let's see if we can figure out who they are." Then list all of the people and animals you encounter while reading the story.
- Close the book and ask your child if she can recall who tried to eat the gingerbread man:
  - The little old man
  - The little old woman
  - The cow
  - The horse
  - The farmers
  - The fox
- After your child has named all the characters that she can remember, open the book and look through the pictures again in sequential order.

Auditory Sequencing

Auditory sequencing enables us to store information that we receive in a meaningful order. It is an important skill that allows us to understand the relationship between the past, the present, and the future and to communicate increasingly complex ideas. Auditory sequencing is a skill that children need in order to grasp the concept of cause and effect. Understanding the relationship between what she sees and why it happened is vital to your child's growing ability to empathize with the emotions on display around her. Suppose your child sees a young girl crying on the playground. She may wonder, "Why is she so sad?" "That little girl is crying because she fell off a swing and hurt her knee," you explain. This simple sequence of cause and effect opens a window that allows your child to compare her emotions with another child's display of feeling. In order to make sense of this information and connect it with what she sees, your child must be able to differentiate between the stages of what happened:

- First, the girl fell off the swing.
- Next, she hurt her knee.
- Last, she started to cry.

Children with an APD often have difficulty making those distinctions and evaluating the information they hear well enough to recall it in sequence. This is why they may have trouble accurately reciting the alphabet, the days of the week, or the months of the year.

You can build your child's auditory sequential memory by asking her to recall the sounds, words, sentences, and events that take place in the following books. Remember to focus on the major events in the story, rather than every detail:

Seven Blind Mice by Ed Young
Chicken Soup with Rice by Maurice Sendak
The Owl and the Pussycat by Edward Lear
Night in the Country by Cynthia Rylant

Auditory Synthesis

Children are not born with the ability to recognize when one sound ends and another begins. They must learn how to discriminate between sequences of speech sounds. It takes years of practice to master this skill. Auditory synthesis is a skill that enables us to smoothly combine sounds or syllables to make a whole word.

You can lay a foundation for your child to become a strong reader and speller by sharing books that offer opportunities to practice listening skills, such as *Sheep Blast Off!* by Nancy Shaw.

Vocabulary

Begin by looking for new words in *Sheep Blast Off!* that your child may not yet understand. Try to use these vocabulary words over the next few days so that your child will become more familiar with any challenging terms:

orbit	panic	blaring	lurch
swoop	hatch	tinker	controls
float	weightless	snoop	explore
	mist		

Explain the double meaning of words your child will encounter in the story: "blast," "touchdown," "seals."

Rhyming

Look for words that rhyme:

tree, be	controls, rolls
stumble, bumble, rumble	gear, stratosphere
last, blast	zips, flips
explore, door, roar	deck, check
okay, way	

Listening to Sounds

Encourage your child to use all of his senses by asking him questions about the kind of sounds he hears in the story.

Thump	"What does a thump sound like?"
	"Can you hear it?"
	"What else makes a thumping sound?"
Rumble	"What does rumble sound like?"
	"Can you hear it?"
	"What else makes a rumbling sound?"
Blare	"What does a blare sound like?"
	"Can you hear it?"
	"What else makes a blaring sound?"
Roar	"What does a roar sound like?"
	"Can you hear it?"
	"What else makes a roaring sound?"

Listening for Sounds

Ask your child to help you find words that begin with certain sounds, such as "sh."

sheep
shape
should

Syllables

Show your child how to clap out the number of syllables he hears in the following words:

One	roar, sheep
Two	landed, stumble
Three	stratosphere

Prosody

It is a good idea to practice changing the sound and the intonation of your voice. This will capture your child's attention and make it more exciting for him to listen. It's also a great way to model how we can effectively use our voices to express different things:

Statement	"Sheep climb through the spaceship door."
Exclamation	"Something has landed!"
Question	"What can it be?"

Action

There are so many wonderful verbs in this book that you can bring to life by acting out their meanings:

Explore	"Let's explore your room and see what we can find."
Jump	"Let's jump like the sheep."
Climb	"Let's climb up the stairs."
Float	"Let's see what will float in the sink."
Grab	"Let's grab our toes."
Press	"Let's press our noses against the window."
Snoop	"Let's snoop under the couch and see what's there."
Bumble	"Let's bumble around the living room."
Tinker	"Let's tinker with your toy and see if we can fix it."

Auditory Memory

After you finish reading the book, ask your child if he remembers some of the events. Look at pictures that appear on the following pages to provide visual cues:

Pages 1–2   "Do you remember which shape the sheep saw?"

             (They saw a spaceship.)

Pages 3–4   "What did the sheep do next?"

             (They climbed through the door in the ship.)

Pages 5–6   "Uh-oh! Do you remember what happened inside the spaceship?"

             (They pushed the buttons and started the ship.)

Retelling

Retelling events that happened in the book will help your child understand sequences. This is a skill your child will need to narrate his own stories and, eventually, to write book reports in school.

You can use ordinal numbers:

First, the sheep saw a spaceship.
Second, the sheep started the spaceship.
Third, the sheep blasted off into space.

Or talk about events that happened:

In the beginning . . .
In the middle . . .
In the end . . .

You can also use transition words:

First, they saw a spaceship.
Then, they started the spaceship.
Next, they blasted off into space.
And then, they were saved by the space alien.
Finally, they landed back on earth.

WHAT TO READ

Sheep Blast Off! is, of course, only one of many good books that you can use to capture a child's imagination while also making listening connections. One of the questions I most often hear from parents is that they are just not sure what to read. They don't know which books will capture their child's attention. While there is no definitive answer, there are a few questions you can ask yourself to find the right book at the right time:

- Is the book funny?
- Does it have interesting vocabulary words?
- Does the book have rhythm and do the words rhyme?
- Does it encourage your child to predict what will happen?
- Does the story relate to something your child is learning at school?
- Does it inspire the imagination?
- Does the book give you something new to talk about?

Reading is also a terrific activity that your whole family can enjoy together. You can read to all of your children at once, even if they are different ages. It is okay to choose a book that is above one child's reading level from time to time, but try not to pick books that are beyond any child's emotional level. This might include stories about illness, war, divorce, death, and other emotionally loaded concepts younger children are not ready to process.

HOW TO READ

Many parents are concerned that they do not have enough time to read every day. But it really only takes a few minutes to enjoy this special time together and to talk about the story:

Currently, Blake loves Dav Pilkey's Captain Underpants books. He can read the text himself but loves it when I read the words to him before bedtime. Blake understands the content and context of the humor and really enjoys the interplay of words in the books. He'll laugh out loud and describe his feelings of enjoyment when we read them together. His articulate appreciation of the books demonstrates that he's moving toward higher levels of critical thinking. As we read together, it's easy to see how far he's come in his oral and aural development, which makes me thank God for Dav Pilkey every day.

—ROSIE

Preschool	Five to ten minutes
Kindergarten	Ten to fifteen minutes
First to third grade	Twenty to thirty minutes

Some children find it difficult to sit still and will get restless after a few minutes. You can build their attention span by gradually increasing the amount of time you spend reading. If your child becomes disinterested in the middle of a book, keep in mind that you don't have to finish a story in one sitting. The quality of the time you spend together is far more important than getting to the end of the book or how many pages you turn.

Try to establish a familiar routine that your child can anticipate and look forward to. It is a good idea to read to your child at the same time each day, whether that is after breakfast, before an afternoon nap, or at bedtime. Even if you can't stick to a regular reading time, make your reading ritual regular and do it together at some point every day.

I encourage parents to create a space for their reading ritual.

Choose a place in your home where your child will be comfortable and cozy and warm. Before reading to your child, you may want to light a candle or sit down on a blanket—anything that separates reading time from the rest of the day and lets her know something special is about to happen.

Invite your child to climb on your lap or sit next to you so that you can establish a shared focus on the book you've chosen and the words and pictures inside. Make sure that the two of you are looking at the book from the same perspective and that your child can easily see the pages. Ask a few simple questions or make comments about what you've just read. These communication checks will let you know if your child is following the story.

Remember to speak slowly and to pause often as you read and talk together. Children must be given a chance to make sense of the information they have just heard and to prepare themselves for more. A moment of silence between thoughts is very powerful, especially for a child with an auditory processing disorder. Pausing gives a child with APD the time she needs to build mental pictures of the story and follow the flow of the narrative.

It is essential that your reading ritual become a rewarding and pleasurable time for both of you, rather than another chore on a long list of things to do. Make sure you're ready to do your part—take a moment to turn off the television, your cell phone, the CD player, and any other distractions so that your environment is more conducive to listening. Never use books as a threat by saying, "If you don't eat your vegetables, you will not get a story tonight," or "If you don't clean your room, we are not going to the library tomorrow."

STORYTELLING

If your child just will not sit still for a book, storytelling can be a magical alternative. This is a completely auditory activity that will help your child build strong listening skills. There are no rules to follow and you can make up stories anywhere. They can be shared in the car, at the dinner table, in a doctor's office, at the beach, or in a park.

Try to stretch your imagination and make believe you are in the midst of a grand adventure with your child. You may find yourselves crawling through the rain forest, climbing a snow-capped mountain, or exploring the depths of the ocean.

Children love to hear stories about their own lives and their family:

- Tell your child about the day she was born.
- Explain how you chose her name.
- Recount things that happened when you were her age, especially stories about things that may be concerning or worrying her, such as the first time you went to school, lost a tooth, rode a bicycle, and so on.
- Talk about your cultural heritage by explaining where your ancestors were born and how they came to live in the United States.
- Share stories about aunts, uncles, grandparents, and great-grandparents to instill a sense of belonging to a larger family.

RECOMMENDED BOOKS FOR EVERY STAGE OF READING

These stories lend themselves beautifully to the kind of listening exercises that we reviewed in this chapter.

Birth to One Year

Goodnight Moon by Margaret Wise Brown is a classic bedtime story that is perfect to share with babies and young children. The tempo of the book is slow and rhythmical, which gives your child time to look at the colorful illustrations. After reading the book together, say good night to some of the things in your child's room as you wave bye-bye.

Listening and Language Activities
- Begin by pointing to and labeling the things you see in the bunny's room: the red balloon, the telephone, the cow jumping over the moon.
- As your child gets older and becomes more familiar with the story, he will start pointing to the pictures when you read the words out loud.
- Your child will soon be able to name on his own all the things he sees in the bunny's room.
- Once your child learns to talk, you can use books to practice rhyming. Try starting a sentence and asking your child to fill in a word that rhymes: "There were three little **bears** sitting in _____." "chairs"

Other Books
> *Black on White* by Tana Hoban
> *Max's First Word* by Rosemary Wells

One to Two Years

Brown Bear, Brown Bear, What Do You See? by Bill Martin, Jr., is another delightful story filled with big pictures of animals on every page. It comes in a board book that is easier for toddlers to handle on their own, as well as a paperback edition.

Listening and Language Activities
- Read the book to your child at least once or twice as you look at the pictures together.

- Then turn the book toward you so that the pages are facing away from your child. "Brown bear, brown bear, what do you see? I see a yellow _____ looking at me." Let your child fill in the animals she remembers seeing. When she responds, flip the book around to show her the picture and confirm, "Yes! It is a yellow duck!" This is such a fun way to build your child's auditory memory as you move through the story.
- Practice coloring pictures of animals and asking, "What does brown bear see?" This will encourage your child to start naming colors and animals as she describes her drawings. "A green pig!"

Other Books
  Rosie's Walk by Pat Hutchins
  Old MacDonald Had a Farm by Colin Hawkins and Jacqui Hawkins
  I Went Walking by Sue Williams

Two to Three Years

The Three Bears by Byron Barton is a simplified version of the classic tale, with brightly colored illustrations.

Listening and Language Activities
  - Talk about the things Goldilocks finds in the bears' house and point out the differences in size. "Look at Papa Bear's *big* chair and Baby Bear's *little* chair."
  - Make size comparisons between objects that you see in your own home: "Look at Daddy's *big* shoe and your *little* shoe."
  - Act out some of the scenes in the book, such as making porridge, setting the table, sitting in chairs, and sleeping in the bed.

Other Books

    Are You My Mother? By P. D. Eastman
    The Three Billy Goats Gruff by Paul Galdone
    Each Peach Pear Plum by Janet and Allan Ahlberg
    Millions of Cats by Wanda Gag
    The Very Hungry Caterpillar by Eric Carle

Three to Four Years

The Snowy Day by Ezra Jack Keats is a beautiful book about wintertime. A little boy named Peter wakes up to find the city he lives in blanketed with snow. He ventures outside to build a snowman and discovers a surprise when he saves a snowball in his pocket.

Listening and Language Activities

- This story lends itself well to a discussion about winter. Make a list of all the things you can do in the snow, such as skiing, skating, snowboarding, sledding, creating snow angels, building snowmen, and so on.
- Cut out photos from a magazine or draw pictures of winter jackets, hats, mittens, boots, and scarves. Make a collage with your child as you talk about the season.
- If you like taking pictures, create your own book of winter experiences featuring images of your child doing fun things in the snow (just like Peter). You can write a simple sentence on each page describing the scene. This little book will become one of your child's most prized possessions. You may be surprised to see how often he looks at it and how much he loves "reading" his own story.

Other Books

    A Color of His Own by Leo Lionni
    If You Give a Mouse a Cookie by Laura Joffe Numeroff

Sam Who Never Forgets by Eve Rice
Sadie and the Snowman by Allen Morgan

Four to Five Years

The Little Red Hen is a classic folktale. Retold by Paul Galdone, this version is set in a barnyard where the little red hen finds a grain of wheat. She asks the cat, the pig, and the duck for help, but none of her friends wants to plant, cut, carry, grind, or bake the wheat into bread.

Listening and Language Activities
- This book has a refrain that encourages children to partici-pate in telling the story. Invite your child to play the part of the lazy friends and shout, "Not I!"

  "Who will help me?" asks the hen.

  "Not I," says the cat.

  "Not I," says the pig.

  "Not I," says the duck.

  "Then I will have to do it myself," says the hen.

Discussion Starters
The story contains a valuable lesson about helping others. If your child is ready to talk about sharing responsibilities, try one of these discussion starters:

"I wonder why the little red hen didn't share her bread with the other animals."

"I wonder what the cat, the pig, and the duck could do next time."

This book naturally leads to a discussion about chores and helping around the house. You can extend the conversation to talk about the importance of picking up toys, clearing the table, putting away clothes, and other tasks.

Other Books
> *Abiyoyo* by Pete Seeger
> *Chrysanthemum* by Kevin Henkes
> *Horton Hatches the Egg* by Dr. Seuss
> *Jack and the Beanstalk* by Paul Galdone

Five to Six Years

Strega Nona, retold by Tomie dePaola, is another classic folktale about a wise woman who has magical powers. Her helper, Big Anthony, causes lots of trouble in the village when he forgets to follow Strega Nona's rules.

Listening and Language Activities
- There is a fun refrain in the book that starts like this:
  > Bubble, bubble, pasta pot
  > Boil me some pasta, nice and hot

  Practice repeating it with your child—and don't forget the three magical kisses at the end!
- Once your child becomes familiar with the story, try beginning the rhyme and ask your child to complete it:
  > Bubble, bubble, pasta ＿＿＿
  > Boil me some pasta, nice and ＿＿＿

Discussion Starters
Strega Nona can teach your child about the importance of listening and following the rules:

"Big Anthony got into a lot of trouble when . . ."
"I wonder what he could have done differently."

"What do you think of Big Anthony's punishment?" (You may have to give your child a hint: he had to eat a town full of pasta.)

Other Books
Alligator Baby by Robert Munsch
Frederick by Leo Lionni
Lentil by Robert McCloskey
Thunder Cake by Patricia Polacco
Wemberly Worried by Kevin Henkes

Six to Seven Years

Cloudy with a Chance of Meatballs by Judi Barrett welcomes your child to the land of Chewandswallow. It is a place where all the food that people want falls from the sky.

Listening and Language Activities
- Can your child imagine how his favorite foods would arrive in Chewandswallow? Would it rain, snow, sleet, or hail?
- Practice naming foods that you serve and describing their flavor.
- Create your own page from the book on a big piece of paper. Ask your child to draw a picture of his favorite food falling from the sky.

Discussion Starters
This is a terrific story that shows your child how too much of a good thing can become a problem.

"I wonder if anything like this could really happen."
"Wouldn't it be great if _____?" (fill in the blank to continue your discussion)

Other Books
    Freckle Juice by Judy Blume
    James and the Giant Peach by Roald Dahl
    Jumanji by Chris Van Allsburg
    Lafcadio, the Lion Who Shot Back by Shel Silverstein

Seven to Eight Years

Your child will begin to enjoy longer books with more text and fewer pictures. *Mr. Popper's Penguins* by Richard and Florence Atwater is a funny old favorite that will lead your child on quite an adventure.

Listening and Language Activities
* Vocabulary. This story is full of words that will build your child's vocabulary: "promptly," "guilty," "customary," "dignity." Look for words that may be new to your child and define what they mean.
* Synonyms. Explain to your child that synonyms are words that mean the same thing. Using clues from the book, try to think of synonyms for the following words: "promptly," "guilty," "customary," and "dignity."

Other Books
    The Cay by Theodore Taylor
    Chocolate Fever by Robert Kimmel Smith
    The Cricket in Times Square by George Selden
    Island of the Blue Dolphins by Scott O'Dell

Reading with Older Children

It is such a joy to spend time sharing stories with children as they grow older. There are many benefits in choosing books that are above your child's own reading level.

- Look for new vocabulary words that appear in the text and talk about what they mean.
- Books allow you to discuss sensitive issues with your child in a more natural and comfortable way.
- Most of all, reading with an older child enables you to stay connected and to share meaningful experiences.

CONTINUING THE STORY

Look for creative ways to bring your child's favorite story to life. There are lots of activities that will extend the enjoyment of a book and make the experience of reading even more memorable.

- Collect objects that appear in the story.
- Draw a picture of a scene in the book.
- Visit the zoo to see some of the animals in the story.
- Prepare one of the meals that characters in the book liked to eat.
- Dramatize one of the events that happened in the story.

BALANCE

There are many books to treasure without the pressure of having to learn a valuable lesson. The most important part of reading with your child is to have fun! Some of the most tender moments that we share with our children happen as we snuggle close together, reading a bedtime story, as our little ones drift off to sleep.

There are many individual books your child will love reading. It may be helpful to refer to these books as well: *The Read-Aloud Handbook* by Jim Trelease, and *Reading Magic: Why Reading Aloud to Our Children Will Change Their Lives Forever* by Mem Fox.

TWELVE

Finding Help

While reading through this book you may have experienced several aha moments—"This sounds like my little boy," or "Oh, I never realized my daughter was struggling with that. No wonder she is so frustrated." You also may have already been focusing on some of the techniques and ideas in this book and are now preparing to recommit to your child's listening well-being based on what you've learned. If you have recognized your child in these pages and want to learn more, then it may be time for you to seek help and begin an evaluation process.

DIAGNOSING APD

In order to adequately assess a child's ability to process auditory information, many of the tests used to diagnose APD require that your child deal with numbers, letters, words, and other ideas and concepts that are out of the reach of younger children. The ability

The parenting journey of discovery can be an intense roller coaster of experiences and emotions. When your child has special needs, that roller coaster has additional loops, whirls, inclines, curves, and steep falls—some scary, some joyful and exciting. The speed of the ride, the jerks and starts, the spins and drops, can be as upsetting as they are invigorating to both parent and child. There are many potential bumps on the road to getting and accepting a child's special needs diagnosis and even more challenges to face when that road widens to include external supports, expert recommendations, and treatment. No matter what diagnosis and what avenue of treatment you, your child, and your support people embark on, it's important to remember that every child is a gift. Your child is a beautiful puzzle that you help put together with the nurturing love and attention that is a parent's greatest strength. Some puzzles are simple, others a little more complicated. But, as parents, we are forever connected to our children, helping to define and strengthen the interlocking pieces that make them who they are, and forming a bigger, clearer picture together.

—ROSIE

to process sound, speech, and language grows over time. Certain specific listening skills such as auditory figure/ground and auditory memory do not develop to a measurable and testable degree in most children until approximately seven years of age. Therefore, APD cannot be definitively diagnosed until around that time. Still, there are professionals and resources that can help you better pinpoint your child's potential issue right from the beginning of his or her life.

FINDING HELP FOR CHILDREN FROM BIRTH TO THREE YEARS OF AGE

If you suspect your child has a speech, language, hearing, or listening problem, which steps to take depend on your child's age.

Ruling Out Hearing Loss

Hearing difficulties in a newborn or infant, such as your child not startling or looking for a loud noise, or failing the universal hearing screening either at birth or when administered a second time, suggest that a hearing test needs to be performed immediately by a pediatric audiologist. Your pediatrician can refer you to an audiologist for this test.

An audiologist is a professional qualified to test hearing and, if a hearing loss is diagnosed, to discuss the level of hearing loss and the best therapy options available. If testing reveals that your child has a measurable hearing loss, an audiologist can provide management services to deal with the problem, including offering a referral for treatment of ear infections or blockages, prescribing hearing aids, or assigning an auditory trainer to give your child extra help. There may be the option of a cochlear implant, depending on the severity of the hearing loss.

Every state has some form of early intervention services to provide help for children from birth to three years of age. Most early intervention services programs can be located and contacted through your local county health department. Your local school district's health service or special needs department can also start you on the way to contacting the right people in your child's school district.

The Next Step: Speech and Language Screening

If a hearing test and examination by an audiologist rules out hearing loss as the source of your child's difficulties, the most likely next step is to arrange a speech and language screening. Children under three years of age are automatically eligible for a speech and language screening by your local early intervention services provider. A speech and language screening will indicate whether your child is experiencing a significant delay in meeting the developmental milestones of speech, language, and listening. If that is the case, your child will then need a speech and language evaluation. The results of the speech and language evaluation will indicate how much and what type of treatment will best suit your child's needs. Keep in mind that each state has different criteria for qualification for intervention services, the types of services available, the frequency with which services are made available (once a week, every day, etc.), where you will need to bring your child for treatment, and the length of time or to what age your child's treatment will remain available.

FINDING HELP FOR CHILDREN AGE THREE THROUGH SCHOOL AGE

If your child is three years of age or older, your local school district is responsible for screening, evaluating, and providing speech, language, and listening intervention. Your child must meet your district's specific criteria and requirements to receive therapy and other special services. The appropriate department within your school district may be called the Committee on Special Education, the Child Study Team, or Pupil Personnel. Contacting your school district office will lead you to the appropriate resources. I know it sounds like a lot to contend with, but remember that the people you contact are there to help. Don't be afraid to ask questions and make as many inquiries as you feel are necessary to have all of your concerns addressed by the service coordinator your state, school, or county health department assigns to your child.

Once hearing loss is ruled out, a speech-language pathologist can evaluate auditory skills and assess if auditory weakness is hindering or slowing your child's speech-language, social, and academic skills development. A speech-language pathologist or speech-language therapist is a professional like me who takes a key role in diagnosing delays and disorders of speech and language acquisition (rather than concentrating primarily on hearing issues, like an audiologist). A speech-language pathologist is qualified to test, diagnose, and treat speech and language delays and disorders.

If speech, language, and listening weaknesses are discovered, the speech-language pathologist can begin intervention and treatment to strengthen areas of auditory weakness, even if your child is too young to be diagnosed with an APD.

WHERE TO GO

Parents and caregivers who suspect that a child of any age may have listening or language skills difficulties have a number of places they can turn to. Some of the organizations, institutions, and groups that offer diagnosis, evaluation, and treatment services for speech-language disorders and APD include:

- Speech-language pathologists in private practice
- Nonprofit social service organizations, such as religious group health initiatives
- Hospitals with speech and language departments
- Universities with speech, language, and audiology clinics

Private, nonprofit social service organizations often provide speech, listening, and language services, evaluation and therapy. Hospitals often have speech and language departments and will provide hearing tests; some may offer a full multidisciplinary evaluation. Universities also often have speech-language and au-diology clinics that will offer screenings, evaluations, and ser-vices.

Your child's pediatrician can be helpful in locating the neces-sary services. Also, the American Speech-Language-Hearing As-sociation (ASHA) has a listing of professionals in your area. A full listing of ASHA contacts by state can be found under Resources at the end of this book. You can also contact ASHA directly at 800–638–8255 or www.asha.org.

Remember that a hearing screening and a hearing evaluation are not the same thing. A hearing screening can be performed by a speech-language pathologist, a school nurse, a physician's assis-tant, or another health professional. Many people, institutions, and organizations offer hearing screenings. A comprehensive as-sessment that narrows down the extent of the hearing loss covers considerably more ground and can only be performed by an au-diologist. Speech and language evaluation is the domain of the speech-language pathologist. Educational testing to rule out or diagnose ADHD, ADD, and other disorders is performed by ed-ucational testing specialists and psychologists.

If by the time your child reaches age seven you believe he is ex-periencing difficulty in auditory processing, APD testing is not the only test to have. A multistage, multidisciplinary assessment is necessary to determine the functional impact of the disorder and to guide treatment and management of APD and associated difficulties. A hearing evaluation followed by a speech-language evaluation will be necessary. While a speech-language pathologist is qualified to gauge the cognitive, communicative, and language factors underlying an APD, not all speech-language pathologists have the same background and expertise. Confirm with your child's evaluator that he or she has had experience evaluating, di-agnosing, and treating children with auditory challenges. In ad-dition, testing by a psychologist may be required as part of the full assessment. After these results are evaluated, the recommendation may be to test for APD.

Testing for APD must be done by an audiologist, but not all audiologists perform APD testing. It is important to find an audiologist with the necessary expertise. When contacting these professionals, whether they work in a doctor's office, private practice, or hospital setting, be sure to confirm that they perform APD testing. For information regarding audiologists in your area, you can contact the American Academy of Audiology, 800-222-2336 or www.audiology.org.

YOU AND YOUR TEAM

Thoroughly diagnosing APD requires input from a team of professionals. An audiologist, an ear-nose-throat specialist, a speech-language pathologist, your child's teachers, social workers, and school or private psychologists are all qualified to contribute to a full APD diagnosis and program of treatment. Once assessments are completed, the team makes recommendations specifically based on your child's performance. These recommendations will be highly individualized and can include:

- Ruling out APD and recommendations for other testing in other areas
- Diagnosis of APD and what areas are affected
- Recommendations for intervention
- Classroom recommendations, such as placement, specific teaching strategies, small-group learning experiences, or physical accommodations within the classroom (preferential seating, amplification such as a personal FM receiver or sound field equipment, or use of noise-dampening techniques). See Chapter 5 for more information on these classroom accommodations.

- Strategies for therapy and treatment
- Short- and long-term goals

QUESTIONNAIRES

There are a number of questionnaires that can be used to help identify children who may benefit from an auditory processing evaluation. Any member of the team of professionals working with you and your child may ask you to provide specific information about your child using a questionnaire. A questionnaire such as any of those listed below gives you the ability to share your observations and knowledge about your child so that the professionals evaluating your child can make comparisons. These questionnaires are valuable tools for gathering information and assessing your child's behavior and abilities in a variety of settings and contexts.

Understanding and helping your child calls for both formal testing and informal observation from you and the professionals you work with. Fact gathering and comparisons made using questionnaires are important because they involve you the parent directly in the evaluation process.

Children's Auditory Processing Performance Scale (CHAPPS)
W. J. Smoski, M. A. Brunt, and J. C. Tanahil (1998)
Educational Audiology Association
11166 Huron Street, Suite 27
Denver, CO 80234
800–460–7322
www.edaud.org

Fisher's Auditory Problems Checklist
L. I. Fisher (1985)
Educational Audiology Association

11166 Huron Street, Suite 27
Denver, CO 80234
800–460–7322
www.edaud.org

The Listening Inventory
D. Geffner and D. Ross-Swain (2006)
Academic Therapy Publications
20 Commercial Boulevard
Novato, CA 94949
800–422–7249
www.academictherapy.com

Getting the correct diagnosis and the right team to support your child as he or she acquires new ways to listen, communicate, and learn is of the utmost importance. Remember that you are the most important member of your child's team. While supporting and advocating for your child, you will in turn need support and guidance yourself to help understand your child's unique way of learning. Finding people who resonate with you, who are helpful, kind, and nonjudgmental while offering you the professional help you and your child need, is very important.

We must remember that our children grow up very quickly and that the intensity of childhood lasts only for a few years. It may seem like a long journey from birth to school age, but the truth is your child's learning style will be set by the time he or she is eight. Those first eight years are a uniquely special time and all too brief.

I hope this book will help you focus on learning as a process and a search for solutions—regardless of the challenges your child may be experiencing—so that you can support each stage of his or her development with the listening and language skills necessary to thrive.

I believe we can fulfill the dreams we have for our children despite the obstacles that may arise along the way.

I believe parents have the power to provide new opportunities for our children to become happier, healthier, wiser, and more compassionate than any other generation.

I know we can raise our sons and daughters with greater awareness, guided by the light of love and wisdom.

I hope this book has given you the inspiration and encouragement you were looking for to help your child listen better, learn better, and live better.

RESOURCES

There are many associations dedicated to the diagnosis and treatment of Auditory Processing Disorder (APD) and other listening, language, and speech disorders. The following list of international, national, state, and local organizations can help you find the professional services and assistance your child may need on his or her path toward success.

INTERNATIONAL

Overseas Association of Communication Sciences (OSACS)
CMR 437, Box 956
APO AE 09267
011–49–621–789–6597

Audiology Online, Inc.
5282 Medical Drive, Suite 150
San Antonio, TX 78229

800–753–2160
210–615–6831
www.audiologyonline.com

NATIONAL

American Speech-Language-Hearing Association (ASHA)
2200 Research Boulevard
Rockville, MD 20850
800–638–8255
www.asha.org

Alexander Graham Bell Association for the Deaf and Hard of Hearing
3417 Volta Place, NW
Washington, DC 20007
202–337–5220
www.agbell.org

Attention Deficit Disorder Association (ADDA)
15000 Commerce Parkway, Suite C
Mount Laurel, NJ 08054
856–439–9099
www.add.org

Autism Society of America
7910 Woodmont Avenue, Suite 300
Bethesda, MD 20814–3067
800–328–8476
301–657–0881
www.autism-society.org

Council for Exceptional Children (CEC)
1110 North Glebe Road, Suite 300
Arlington, VA 22201
703–620–3660
www.cec.sped.org

Council for Learning Disabilities (CLD)
11184 Antioch Road, #405
Overland Park, KS 66210
913–491–1011
www.cldinternational.org

National Center for Learning Disabilities (NCLD)
381 Park Avenue South, Suite 1401
New York, NY 10016
212–545–7510
www.ld.org

National Coalition on Auditory Processing Disorders
www.ncapd.org

National Dissemination Center for Children with Disabilities (NICHCY)
P.O. Box 1492
Washington, DC 20013–1492
202–884–8200
www.nichcy.org

National Institute on Deafness and Other Communication Disorders (NIDCD)
31 Center Drive, MSC 2320
Bethesda, MD 20892–2320

800–241–1044
301–496–7243
www.nidcd.nih.gov

National Organization for Hearing Research Foundation (NOHR)
225 Haverford Avenue, Suite 1
Narberth, PA 19072–2234
610–664–3135
www.nohrfoundation.org

National Resource Center on AD/HD
8181 Professional Place, Suite 150
Landover, MD 20785
800–233–4050
www.help4adhd.org

STATE

Speech and Hearing Association of Alabama
P.O. Box 130220
Birmingham, AL 35213
205–802–7551
www.alabamashaa.org

Alaska Speech-Language-Hearing Association
P.O. Box 568
Kodiak, AK 99615
907–486–9132
www.aksha.org

Arizona Speech-Language-Hearing Association
P.O. Box 30988
Phoenix, AZ 85046

602–354–8062
www.arsha.org

Arkansas Speech-Language-Hearing Association
Martinsen Management
P.O. Box 250261
Little Rock, AR 72225–0261
501–244–0261
www.arksha.org

California Speech-Language-Hearing Association
825 University Avenue
Sacramento, CA 95825
916–921–1568
www.csha.org

Colorado Speech-Language-Hearing Association
P.O. Box 345
Sedalia, CO 80135–0345
720–733–9097
www.cshassoc.org

Connecticut Speech-Language-Hearing Association, Inc.
213 Back Lane
Newington, CT 06111–4204
860–666–6900
www.ctspeechhearing.org

Delaware Speech-Language-Hearing Association, Inc.
P.O. Box 7383
Newark, DE 19711
www.dsha.org

District of Columbia Speech-Language-Hearing Association
P.O. Box 29590
Washington, DC 20017
202–269–7666
www.dcsha.org

Florida Association of Speech-Language Pathologists and Audiologists
222 South Westmonte Drive, Suite 101
Altamonte Springs, FL 32714
800–243–3574
www.flasha.org

Georgia Speech-Language-Hearing Association
2020 Howell Mill Road, Suite C-295
Atlanta, GA 30318
800–226–4742
http://web.memberclicks.com/mc/page.do?orgId=gsa

Hawaii Speech-Language-Hearing Association
P.O. Box 235888
Honolulu, HI 96823–3514
www.hsha.org

Idaho Speech, Language and Hearing Association, Inc.
1411 East Amity Avenue
Nampa, ID 83686–5540
208–467–4829
www.idahosha.org

Illinois Speech-Language-Hearing Association
230 East Ohio Street, Suite 400
Chicago, IL 60611–3265

312–644–0828
www.ishail.org

Indiana Speech-Language-Hearing Association
1829 Conningham Road
Indianapolis, IN 46224
317–916–4146
www.islha.org

Iowa Speech-Language-Hearing Association
Diversified Management Services (ISHA)
525 S.W. Fifth Street, Suite A
Des Moines, IA 50309
515–282–8192
www.isha.org

Kansas Speech-Language-Hearing Association
6001 Cherokee Drive
Fairway, KS 66205
913–362–0015
www.ksha.org

Kentucky Speech-Language-Hearing Association
535 West Second Street, Suite 103
Lexington, KY 40508
859–252–3776
www.kysha.org

Louisiana Speech-Language-Hearing Association
8550 United Plaza Boulevard, Suite 1001
Baton Rouge, LA 70809
225–922–4512
www.lsha.org

Maine Speech-Language-Hearing Association
P.O. Box 367
Strong, ME 04983
207–338–9349
www.mslha.org

Maryland Speech-Language-Hearing Association
P.O. Box 31
Manchester, MD 21102
410–239–7770
www.mdslha.org

Massachusetts Speech-Language-Hearing Association
411 Waverly Oaks Road, Suite 331B
Waltham, MA 02452
781–647–7031
www.mshahearsay.org

Michigan Speech-Language-Hearing Association
790 West Lake Lansing Road, Suite 500-A
East Lansing, MI 48823
517–332–5691
www.michiganspeechhearing.org

Minnesota Speech-Language-Hearing Association
1821 University Avenue West, Suite S256
St. Paul, MN 55104
651–999–5350
www.msha.net

Mississippi Speech-Language-Hearing Association
P.O. Box 22664
Jackson, MS 39225–2664

800–664–6742

www.mshausa.org

Missouri Speech-Language-Hearing Association

2000 East Broadway, PMB 296

Columbia, MO 65201

888–729–6742

www.showmemsha.org

Montana Speech, Language and Hearing Association

P.O. Box 215

Miles City, MT 59301

406–234–8727

www.mshaonline.org

Nebraska Speech-Language-Hearing Association

455 South 11th Street, Suite A

Lincoln, NE 68508–2105

402–476–9573

www.nslha.org

Nevada Speech-Language-Hearing Association

P.O. Box 7313

Reno, NV 89510–7313

775–851–7166

www.nvsha.org

New Hampshire Speech-Language-Hearing Association, Inc.

P.O. Box 1538

Concord, NH 03302–1538

603–228–5949

www.nhslha.org

New Jersey Speech-Language-Hearing Association
203 Towne Centre Drive
Hillsborough, NJ 08844
908–534–4879
www.njsha.org

New Mexico Speech and Hearing Association
P.O. Box 66085
Albuquerque, NM 87193–3580
505–899–6674
www.nmsha.net

New York State Speech-Language-Hearing Association, Inc.
1 Northway Lane
Latham, NY 12110
518–786–0947
www.nysslha.org

North Carolina Speech-Language-Hearing Association
P.O. Box 28359
Raleigh, NC 27611–8359
919–833–3984
www.ncshla.org

North Dakota Speech-Language-Hearing Association
P.O. Box 12775
Grand Forks, ND 58208–2775
701–780–2439
www.minotstateu.edu/ndslha

Ohio Speech-Language-Hearing Association
P.O. Box 309
Germantown, OH 45327–0309

800–866-OSHA
www.ohioslha.org

Oklahoma Speech-Language-Hearing Association
P.O. Box 890059
Oklahoma City, OK 73189–0059
405–664–3715
www.oslha.org

The Oregon Speech-Language-Hearing Association
P.O. Box 523
Salem, OR 97308
503–370–7019
www.oregonspeechandhearing.org

Pennsylvania Speech-Language-Hearing Association
800 Perry Highway, Suite 3
Pittsburgh, PA 15229–1128
412–366–9858
www.psha.org

Rhode Island Speech-Language-Hearing Association
P.O. Box 9241
Providence, RI 02940
401–455–7472
www.risha.info

South Carolina Speech-Language-Hearing Association
701 Gervais Street, Suite 150–206
Columbia, SC 29201
888–729–3717
www.scsha.com

South Dakota Speech-Language-Hearing Association
P.O. Box 308
Sioux Falls, SD 57101–0308
605–274–2423
www.sdslha.org

Tennessee Association of Audiology and Speech-Language Pathology
P.O. Box 331307
Nashville, TN 37203–7513
615–528–9021
www.taaslp.org

Texas Speech-Language-Hearing Association
918 Congress Avenue, Suite 200
Austin, TX 78701
512–494–1127
www.txsha.org

Utah Speech-Language-Hearing Association
P.O. Box 3074
Salt Lake City, UT 84110–3074
435–797–7554
www.ushaonline.net

Vermont Speech-Language-Hearing Association, Inc.
2 Southwind Drive
Brownsville, VT 05037
www.vsha.us

Speech-Language-Hearing Association of Virginia, Inc.
3126 West Cary Street, #436
Richmond, VA 23221

888–729–7428
www.shav.org

Washington Speech and Hearing Association
2150 North 107th Street, Suite 205
Seattle, WA 98133
206–367–8704
www.wslha.org

West Virginia Speech-Language-Hearing Association
941 Farms Drive
Fairmont, WV 26554
www.wvsha.org

**Wisconsin Speech-Language Pathology and Audiology
Professional Association**
P.O. Box 1109
Madison, WI 53701
608–283–5489
www.wisha.org

Wyoming Speech-Language-Hearing Association
760 West 57th Street
Casper, WY 82601
307–265–1166
www.wsha.info

SELECTED REFERENCES
AND BIBLIOGRAPHY

ASHA. 2005. Central auditory processing disorders—the role of the audiologist. American Speech-Language-Hearing Association. Retrieved from www.asha.org/docs/html/PS2005–00114.html.

Bellis, Teri James. 2002. *When the Brain Can't Hear: Unraveling the Mystery of Auditory Processing Disorder.* New York: Atria Books.

Bloom, L., and M. Lahey. 1978. *Language Development and Language Disorders.* New York: John Wiley and Sons.

Calkins, Lucy McCormick. 2001. *The Art of Teaching Reading.* New York: Addison-Wesley.

Duchan, J. F., and J. Katz. 1983. Language and auditory processing: top down plus bottom up. In E. Z. Laskey and J. Katz (Eds.), *Central Auditory Disorders: Problems of Speech, Language and Learning.* Baltimore, MD: University Park Press.

Elkind, David. 2007. *The Power of Play.* New York: DaCapo Press.

Erber, N. P. 1982. *Auditory Training.* Washington, DC: Alexander Graham Bell Association for the Deaf.

Flexer, Carol. 1994. *Facilitating Hearing and Listening in Young Children.* San Diego, CA: Singular Publishing Group, Inc.

Gillet, P. 1993. *Auditory Processes*. Novato, CA: Academic Therapy Publications.

Ginott, H. G. 1965, 2003. *Between Parent and Child*. New York: Three Rivers Press.

Greenspan, S., and S. Wieder. 1998. *The Child with Special Needs: Encouraging Intellectual and Emotional Growth*. Cambridge, MA: Perseus Publishing.

Healy, J. 1990. *Endangered Minds: Why Our Children Can't Think*. New York: Simon and Schuster.

Healy, Jane M. 1987. *Your Child's Growing Mind*. New York: Simon and Schuster.

Kelly, Dorothy A. 1995. *Central Auditory Processing Disorder: Strategies for Use with Children and Adolescents*. San Antonio, TX: Communication Skill Builders.

Levitan, D. 2006. *This Is Your Brain on Music*. New York: Dutton.

Luria, A. R. 1982. *Language and Cognition*. New York: John Wiley.

Madule, Paul. 1993. *When Listening Comes Alive*. Norval, ON: Moulin Publishing.

Rawson, Martyn, and Michael Rose. 2002. *Ready to Learn: From Birth to School Readiness*. Gloucestershire, UK: Hawthorn Press.

Richard, Gail. 2001. *The Source for Processing Disorders*. East Moline, IL: LinguiSystems.

Smaldino, J., and C. Crandell. Classroom amplification technology: theory and practice. *Lang. Sp. Hear. Serv. Schools* 2000(31):371–375.

Trelease, J. 1982. *The Read Aloud Handbook*. New York: Penguin Books.

Vygotsky, L. S. 1962. *Thought and Language*. Cambridge, MA: MIT Press.

Zigler, E., D. Singer, and S. Bishop-Joseph. 2004. *Children's Play: The Roots of Reading*. Washington, DC: Zero to Three Press.

ACKNOWLEDGMENTS

I believe we do not travel through life alone. I am so grateful to the wonderful people in my life who have had a profound effect on me. They have served as mentors, friends, loved ones, and supporters.

I feel so fortunate to be working with my literary agents, Shawn Coyne and Richard Abate; my editor, Marnie Cochran; my friend Ed O'Donnell.

My life has been enriched by my mentors, Connie Carlough, David Luterman, and Nancy Cooke de Herrera, who have pointed me in the right direction at important crossroads in my life; my husband, Peter, my strongest supporter and love; my children, Isaac and Gabriel, whom I once guided and who now guide me; my sister, Susan, who has always been beside me.

And Rosie O'Donnell, who believes that we need to help all children reach their true potential, and who has given me the opportunity to share my life's work through this book.

With love, I thank you all.

INDEX